THE ESSENTIALS OF EMERGENCY PREPAREDNESS

A PRIMER FOR HEALTHCARE PROVIDERS

Thomas Calhoun MD, MS, FACN, FACS

author**HOUSE**

AuthorHouse™
1663 Liberty Drive
Bloomington, IN 47403
www.authorhouse.com
Phone: 833-262-8899

Published by AuthorHouse 10/30/2024

ISBN: 979-8-8230-1785-5 (sc)
ISBN: 979-8-8230-1784-8 (e)

Library of Congress Control Number: 2023922064

Dedicated to my wife Shirley, who is her quiet, subtle way would often say/ask, "It's nice that you have finished your other Books, but what about the one on Emergency Preparedness, I think that's the one people need"?

The views expressed in this book are solely the work of the author, with the material noted in the quotes ("..."), all having been meticulously searched for and reviewed for accuracy.

With the constant changing of the Internet, any links and web addresses listed here-in, may well have changed, or no longer exist, since this book was started in 2008.

I would like to thank my brother, William. M Thompson, PhD, Clinical Psychology, and his wife Mary, for their assistance in writing Chapter 12, and my sister-in-law, Margaret Jones Woody for designing the cover for the book.

"We have grasped the mystery of the atom and rejected the Sermon on the Mount".

Omar Bradley

CONTENTS

Chapter 5

Chapter 6 A

Chapter 6 B

FOREWORD

It was a busy Thursday afternoon, around rush hour, and numerous healthcare providers offices were filled with patients.

Suddenly, TV`s in the waiting rooms interrupt their usual programs with breaking news; "The Mayor has just indicated that a Dirty Bomb has exploded in the middle of down town, and he has issued an order that all facilities and residents must "Shelter in place"!

There is a stir in the waiting rooms and in a trice, as if with one voice, there is a question from the waiting room, "Are we going to die"?

So what is the healthcare providers' response?

Given the current state of world affairs, healthcare providers should be prepared, or are preparing for how to respond to any All-Hazardous Emergency if/when called upon.

This Book is a handy reference to help those providers respond in a calm, professional manner, whether in the private office setting, or to the local Department of Health, which may reach out for assistance.

Accompanying this Book also, are 101 questions and answers, which the Academic community can use in conjunction with their Mission in training competent professionals to confront these issues.

PREFACE

On Wednesday October 17, 2001, about 3:30 pm, I received a phone call from the Chief Operating Officer of the Delmarva Foundation for Medical Care, the Professional Review Organization (PRO), for the State of Maryland and the District of Columbia (DC). At the time I was the Medical Director for the DC PRO.

The charge, find out what information Physicians in the District of Columbia needed about Anthrax.

It was on October 9, 2001 that a letter containing Anthrax spores had been mailed to the office of a United States Senator and eventually opened by the Senator's staff 6 days later. By October 30, 2001, 5 individuals who worked at the Brentwood United States (US) Postal facility would be hospitalized at local hospitals, 2 of whom would die, one within 5 days of the onset of symptoms, one within 7 days. [1a]

This mandate was going out nation-wide from the Healthcare Finance Administration (HCFA) to all 50 PROs`, representing all 50 States and the District of Columbia, and responses were expected by close of business on Friday, October 17, 2001.

HCFA is now the Centers for Medicare and Medicaid Services (CMS).

A phone call went out from my office to various Chairs of Departments of Medicine and Surgery whom I knew in the DC area, asking for help. By mid-day on Thursday, October 18, I had input from a number of individuals and I prepared a one-page list of 5 questions

(Unfortunately I did not retain a copy of those questions) which I passed out at the quarterly Medical Staff meeting which was held at Providence Hospital here in DC the following Thursday evening.

This very unscientific approach resulted in the collective statement, "I need as much information as possible and as soon as possible"!

That week-end, I was one of the volunteer physicians who provided prophylactic antibiotics to the approximately 30, 000 individuals who presented themselves at the old DC General Hospital in Southeast Washington.

These were individuals who were exposed, or thought they were exposed to the Anthrax.

Other than the two Post Office employees who died, as noted above, no other cases of Anthrax were discovered in the District of Columbia.

In March, 2003, I began work in the Emergency Health and Medical Administration (EHMSA) for the DC Department of Health as the first Medical Director for Bioterrorism. Later I would be named Interim Administrator for EHMSA.

In this position, along with the Director of the DC Department of Health, I attended multiple medical and community meetings, discussing various aspects of Bioterrorism, which following the Anthrax event, along with the September 11, 2001 terrorists' bombings, had resulted in Emergency Preparedness becoming the number one health and safety issue in the country.

Personally, I would be vaccinated with the Small pox vaccine March 17, 2003. I recall having been previously vaccinated at a young age, perhaps 9 or 10, at St. Pius Catholic School in Jacksonville, Florida.

As best I can recall, at that time all of us stayed in school and had no concerns about Small pox or the vaccine; nor did the Teachers or our parents, I think, not knowing anything about complications of the vaccine.

Now, there are specific criteria for who should be vaccinated in a pre-event Small pox outbreak which will be discussed later.

Age was a risk factor for being vaccinated. I was 71 years old but I had no complications from the vaccine.

A few years later, May 18, 2007, I would receive a Master's of Science Degree in Bio-hazardous Threat Agents and Emerging Infectious Diseases from Georgetown University here in the District of Columbia, and the seed for my writing this book was sewn.

In part, because of my own interests and experiences as Medical Director and interacting with various healthcare providers in many disciplines, it became very clear to me that there was a dearth of information on Emergency Preparedness available in one easily read document for the busy healthcare professional, not directly associated with Emergency Preparedness.

This was again brought to mind while attending the National Medical Association's annual meeting in Las Vegas, Nevada, in August, 2009.

A representative from the CDC was presenting information on the H_1N_1 Influenza and one of the Physicians from the audience asked if there was a document available with information on Emergency Preparedness?

The response was that one could go to the CDC website for information.

At that moment, I knew as a practicing Physician myself, that the average Physician would not have the time, nor inclination, to go on line to look for information if an emergency arose, and they were in an Office setting with numerous patients.

The need, in my opinion, was a single document which could be used as a quick reference and which covers in a general sense, the broad area of Emergency Preparedness.

I, the Author, do not in any way intend to imply that I am an expert, of any sort, but am writing material which is in the literature, and which I have meticulously searched for and quoted.

Accompanying the book is a set of 101 questions and answers for those who would choose to become more thoroughly grounded in Emergency Preparedness, and which can be used in conjunction with this book for the students at the undergraduate or graduate level.

The information presented here-in is entirely within the public domain in some format, and this is an attempt to present in organized form, what should be an efficient approach to aid in recognizing threats from the agents described, and an appropriate response from the healthcare provider.

Moreover, the healthcare provider would understand the collaborative role they may have with local, state and federal agencies should they become a part of the disaster.

Indeed, in an article in the Journal of the American Medical Association (JAMA) dated February 20, 2002 [1b] entitled "Bioterrorism Preparedness and Response: Clinicians and Public Health Agencies as Essential Partners", the authors discuss the multiple medical specialties involved in the response to the intentional distribution of the Bacillus anthracis spores through the postal system. The article notes that "22 individuals were infected with 5 deaths from the infection". This resulted in some 30,000 individuals being given prophylactic antibiotics here in the District of Columbia, the Author being one of the physicians providing the antibiotics.

It should be paramount in the providers' thought process that self-protection and prudence must prevail when dealing with a disaster.

If those who have some degree of training and expertise become compromised, they may well become a liability to more than themselves.

This response is further emphasized later in the discussion on "Situation awareness".

For all who may have the occasion to read this Primer, a major feature of your involvement should be participating in and or strongly recommending frequent preparedness exercises and All-hazards drills, not just Fire drills.

As the country has moved farther away from the initial event in October 2001, the desire and will to participate in many Table-Top Exercises and full-scale Exercises appears to have been lacking, at least as recognized by large scale press coverage.

It is not a small undertaking to practice and actually evacuate an office or clinic or building, but if this has not occurred, with a safe secondary site for relocation, when the actual emergency occurs, that will become much more problematic.

The following are some common terms which may be associated with Emergency Preparedness:

Emergency-an event which may result in physical property destruction and or injury, with possible loss of life or limb. These events usually will not exceed local emergency response capability.

Cataclysm- the same as a disaster but exceeds all response capacity, e.g., the massive earthquakes in China where 255,000 were killed in 1976, Indonesia in 2004, triggering the tsunami which killed 228,000 and the earthquake in Haiti, 2010 with the estimated death toll of over 200,000. [2]

Critical Incident- a generally unexpected challenging event with the potential for causing significant human distress. The response may create new positive growth as the region may be forced to interact with local, state or federal agencies.

Disaster- an unplanned or unexpected event that results in a large amount of physical destruction, injury, loss of life and a high degree of social disruption, which usually exceeds local emergency response capability.

(Hurricanes Katrina in New Orleans, Rita in Mississippi, August 2005, and Ike in Galveston and Houston, September 2008).

Endemic- "The habitual presence of a disease within a given geographic area". [3]

Epidemic- "The occurrence in a community or region of a group of illnesses of similar nature, clearly in excess of normal expectancy, and derived from a common, or from a propagated source".

Pandemic "refers to a world-wide epidemic". [3]

Terrorism-as defined by Law Enforcement is the premeditated and unlawful use or threat of force or violence as a punitive or coercive measure.

As defined by the Military it is war or military action against civilians or non-combatants.

As defined in the Healthcare community, it is a psychological or behavioral tool with the goal to create fear and helplessness and to break down resistance or the will of the population or its government.

An example of this is Russia's current bombing of schools and hospitals in Ukraine.

Post-Traumatic Stress (PTS) - a normal behavioral survival response, generally requires no significant long term healthcare input.

Post-Traumatic Stress Disorder (PTSD)-an abnormal or pathological variant of the normal behavioral survival response and may require significant long term healthcare intervention.

Herd Immunity-the resistance of a group to an attack by a disease to which large numbers of the group have been vaccinated, or were previously infected, and are immune. [3]

Incubation Period-the interval of time from which an infection occurs to the time of onset of clinical illness. [3]

Attack Rate-the number of people at risk, who develop a particular illness, divided by the total number of people at risk, multiplied by 100.

Case Fatality Rate-the number of individuals dying during a specified period of time after disease onset, or diagnosis divided by the number of individuals with the disease, multiplied by 100.

Incidence-(of a disease)-the number of new cases that occur during a specified period of time, in a population at risk for developing the disease during that period of time, multiplied by 1,000.

Prevalence-the number of affected persons present in the population at a specific time, divided by the number of persons in the population at that specified time, multiplied by 1,000.

RADAR-Radio and Detection and Ranging.

LASER-Light Amplification by the Stimulated Emission of Radiation.

[1a.] DA Henderson, TV Inglesby, T O` Toole, Bioterrorism: Guidelines for Medical and Public Health Management, JAMA Archives Journals 2002.
[1b.] Gerberding, J, Hughes, J, Koplan, J, Bioterrorism Preparedness and Response: Clinicians and Public Health Agencies as Essential Partners, JAMA, Feb., 2002, Vol 287, No 7:897-900; see also pp 857-874.
[2.] The Washington Post, p A10, February 28, 2010.
[3.] Epidemiology, 2nd ed., Leon Gordis, W.B. Saunders Co. 2000, Chapters 2 and 3.

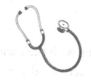

CHAPTER 1

INCIDENT MANAGEMENT SYSTEM (IMS)

INCIDENT COMMAND SYSTEM (ICS)
LEGAL ISSUES

"Never mistake motion for action."

Ernst Hemingway

A. Structure:

1. Incident Commander
        Public Information Officer
        Safety Officer
        Liaison Officer
2. Operations officer
3. Planning Officer (PI)
4. Logistics Officer
5. Administration Officer

B. Functions:

Incident Commander – has overall authority for managing the incident; delegates as needed.

Public Information Officer – coordinates all media activities with the Incident Commander.

Safety Officer – coordinate safety activities, develops safety plan.

Has the authority, along with the Incident Commander to temporarily abort any activity deemed unsafe.

Liaison Officer – primary contact to, and from, other agencies involved in the incident allowing for concurrent interchange of information, in addition to telephones, e-mail and faxes.

Planning Officer – provided technical advice, coordinates resource utilization, along with Incident Commander, prepares incident action (an After Action) plan.

Operations Officer – coordinates operational strategy, fire and rescue. Health and Emergency Medical Services (EMS), law enforcement activities may involve ground and air resources.

Administration Officer – coordinates accurate and detailed documentation of activities, time, costs, compensation, and claims.

Note: Each section has adequate personnel, communication, and equipment for performing functions.

The Safety Officer (and staff) is alerted to prevent "Burn Out" at any position along the incident management/command system.

(This schema and structure have been updated. See references below).

A thorough understanding of the ICS offers the best opportunity for responding to a major disaster with the expectation of a successful outcome.

The Incident Command System evolved from experiences in the Fire Department in the State of California.

It is a coordinated strategy using a common nomenclature with all of the participants buying into the concept.

One individual is in charge at all times, located in a Command Center, from which all activities are coordinated.

Each of the 8 individuals in the Command Structure has specific responsibilities, with appropriately trained back-up, for timely relief.

The depth of the structure depends upon the disaster, the size of the organization and the duration of the event, which initially is likely unknown.

The system needs to be practiced on a regular basis, to include back up personnel, communication systems and coordination with the next higher level of Command, e.g., Public Health Agencies.

The disaster may require a Unified Command Structure, for example, a chemical event, which would require a Hazardous Unit from the Fire Department, and Healthcare personnel from the Department of Health.

In this context a Joint Information Center (JIC) should be established which will allow for better coordination of information.

For a detailed review of the Incident Management System, refer to:

> Response – field guide for Fire and EMS Organizations:
> Paul M. Maniscol, MPA, PhD, EMT/D, Hank
> T. Christen, MPA EMT/B (Prentice Hall), 20003

Hospital Emergency Incident Command System (HEICS)

This form of the Incident Command System was developed in hospitals in Orange County, California in 1991. Based on the ICS model, it defines responsibilities, uses prioritized check lists, has clear reporting channels and management structure and utilizes a common nomenclature which helps unify the Hospital and other emergency disaster responders.

> (California Emergency Medical Services
> Authority, Hospital Emergency Incident
> Command System III, Project 2003).

Note, the schema and or functions of these organizations may have changed since we began writing this book.

Legal Issues.

In the aftermath of 911 and the Anthrax incident in 20011, the need for better preparation and coordination of resources became readily evident to Federal, State and Local leaders.

On the National level the Office of Homeland Security within the Executive Office of the President, headed by former Pennsylvania Governor Tom Ridge, was created.

Congress would pass several important Acts addressing many of these issues. [1]

The Aviation and Transportation Security Act established a federal agency to supervise security of commercial aviation. The Maritime Transportation

Security Act instituted new requirements for the security of ports and shipping.

The Enhanced Border Security and Visa Entry Reform Act increased information requirements from visitors to the United States.

The Public Health Security and Bioterrorism Preparedness and Response Act required additional protections for the food and drug supply.

One of the most important Acts to be passed was the USA PATRIOT Act- Providing Appropriate Tools Required to Intercept and Obstruct Terrorism. *

The Act created new crimes, penalties and efficient procedures to be used against international and domestic terrorists. This would be accomplished by promoting sharing information between law enforcement and intelligence agencies; authorizing other law enforcement tools which were already available for pursing drug smuggling and other serious crimes, and improved surveillance of terrorist by using new technologies such as cell phones and the Internet.

Further, it provided for congressional and judicial oversight of the new authorities.

There were unintended consequences of the Act however; reduced public accountability, allowing government officials to target citizens not under criminal investigation and allowing unlawful imprisonment.

*https://www.britannica.com>topic>USA-PATRIOT-Act, USA

PATRIOT ACT| Facts, History, Acronym & Controversy| Britannica.

The Homeland Security Presidential Directive #5 required, via the National Incident Management System the standardization of Incident Management for All Hazards, with appropriate instruction for the Incident Command System and the Unified Command where needed.

For a more in-depth review of additional legislative measures following 911 and Anthrax in 2001, see reference [1] below, from which much of the above information was taken.

The role of the Military in providing support to civil authorities in cases of major disaster or terrorism in the United States or its territories deserves noting.

In 1878 the Posse Comitatus Act which prohibited federal troops from enforcing state or federal laws without congressional approval was passed (1 p 8). This came about after President Rutherford B. Hayes sent troops to the polling stations in Florida, South Carolina and Louisiana due to the continuing dispute about the electoral votes in 1876. Over time with the passage of other Acts, e.g., the Stafford Act [3] did allow for the Department of Defense (DOD) to provide support for civilian agencies. Currently Posse Comitatus prohibits federal forces from performing law enforcement activities without congressional permission. Training of civil authorities, logistical support, technical advice and equipment loans can be provided.

In 1996 after a review of US capabilities to respond to Weapons of Mass Destruction (WMD), specifically Chemical and Biological agents, the Department of Defense was required by congress to provide training in these areas to local and State officials who would act as First Responders in the event of a terrorist event. [2]

Moreover, the DOD was authorized to support the Department of Justice in their law enforcement activities in emergencies involving chemical and biological agents used as WMDs, which is an exception to the Posse Comitatus Act.

1.2 Sauter, M, Carafano, JJ, A Complete Guide to Understanding, Preventing and Surviving Terrorism, Homeland Security, Chapter 3, pp 41-59, 2005, McGraw Hill.

1. Smith, J, Thomas, WC, The Terrorism Threat and US Government Response: Operational and Organizational Factors, Chapter

10, INSS Book Series, 2001 http://www.usafa.edu/df/inss/terrorism.htm

2. The Robert T. Stafford Disaster Relief and Emergency Assistance Act (Pub. Law 100-707).

Allows for the President to declare an emergency, amended in 1988 which activates financial and physical responses from the Federal Emergency Management Agency (FEMA), to coordinate government wide relief efforts. Responses were through the Federal Response Plan, now National Response Plan. The Act was amended in 2000 with the passage of the Disaster Mitigation Act (Pub.L.106-390) and again in 2006 with the Pets Evacuation and Transportation Standards Act (Pub.L.109-308). http://en.wikipedia.org/wiki/Stafford_Act

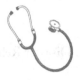

CHAPTER 2

PERSONAL PROTECTIVE EQUIPMENT (PPE)

"By his deeds we know a man".

African Proverb

A basic understanding and familiarity with Personal Protective Equipment is essential for the Healthcare provider and for those who may be called upon as first responders. Preparations for Chemical, Biological, Radiological, Nuclear or Explosive Agents (CBRNE) will be very helpful for responding to Natural disasters.

Preparations include breathing equipment, gloves, gowns, goggles, face shields, equipment needed to successfully address these situations. It is important that the Healthcare provider not undertake any hazardous situation he or she is not trained for. The proper use of PPE will help prevent transferring hazardous material from infected individuals and an unsafe environment to the Healthcare worker and or the unaffected individual.

Aside from a direct explosion, the common routes of exposure are inhalation, ingestion, via the skin and eyes, or infection. Chemical agents' exposure may occur via inhalation of a gas or vapor. The eyes and skin may have direct contact from vapors or liquid. Inhalation of biological agents as droplets or aerosols is the most common route of exposure. Ingestion of agents from food or liquids is a common occurrence also, whereas generally the intact skin is not; exceptions being Mustard Gas and Fires.

Agents can be injected as in the classic case of Gregor Markov who was injected "accidentally" via an umbrella. If there is an explosion or fire, individuals can become contaminated with radio-active material, as could be the case from a "Dirty Bomb – Radio-active Diversion Device (RDD)." In these settings clothing, hair, skin, eyes, may become contaminated.

Internal contamination may occur from ingesting radio-active material and inhalation of highly radioactive dust particles could occur. In all of these situations, the goal is to prevent contamination from the victim to the rescue or treatment individual.

Healthcare workers, for whom this Primer is intended, generally will not require high levels of PPE, unless they are involved as First Responders.

Surgical Masks –protects the clean/sterile field of the patient and provides some protection for the Healthcare provider - they offer no respiratory protection from chemicals, but are effective against respiratory droplets such as from Influenza or pneumonic plague.

N-95 Masks, N-100 Masks –these filter 95 and 100 percent respectively, droplets of airborne biological aerosols, and should be worn by the Healthcare workers as the incident dictates.

These require fit-testing on periodic basis as prescribed by the Occupational Safety and Health Administration (OSHA).

In the event of a Pandemic, this requirement may be changed.

Another protective respiratory device is the Self-Contained Breathing Apparatus (SCBA). An open circuit positive – pressure apparatus provides the highest level of respiratory protection.

Supplied Air Respirator (SAR) – less bulky than SCBA, also provides the highest level of respiratory protection. Air Purifying Respirators (APR) are of the disposable and chemical types.

Disposal APRs which do not provide eye protection, are enhanced however, when used in combination with a high efficiency particulate filter and chemical cartridge. A Powered Air Purifying Respirator (PAPR) may be required.

Chemical Cartridges (canisters) are effective against various gases and vapors. High-efficiency particulate air filters (HEPA) are effective in the 98-100% range in excluding highly infections particles in the 1 to 5 micro meter range, such as for Small pox or the viral Hemorrhagic fever or Severe, Acute Respiratory Syndrome (SARS).

The N-95 Mask was highly effective in the SARS outbreak in 2003. Healthcare workers are generally familiar with the usual precautions of gown, gloves, and hoods, face shield in dealing with contaminated or isolated patients.

Always wash the hands with soap and water or alcohol-based hand sanitizer, before and after tending the contaminated or isolated patient.

Civilian Personal Protection Equipment is designated by the U.S. Environmental Protection Agency (EPA) into 4 levels:

Level A – SCBA, a totally encapsulating chemical protective outfit that provides the highest level of respiratory, eye, mucus membrane and skin protection.

Level B – a positive pressure respirator (SCBA or SAR) and incomplete covering of garments, gloves and boots, provides respiratory protection and a lower level of skin protection.

Level C –Air Purified Respirator an incomplete covering of chemical resistant clothes, gloves and boots; same level of skin protection as Level

B but lower level of respiratory protection. The type of airborne exposure is known and guarded against for Level C exposure.

Level D – Standard work clothes without a respirator – generally the hood, gown, mask, latex gloves (or non-allergenic) – or universal precautions (now referred to as standard precautions), minimal skin and respiratory protection provided under the N-95, N-100 Masks used.

Often the offending agent(s) is/are unknown initially and to allow for proper decontamination and the safety of the healthcare workers, triage teams designate "zones" of involvement.

Hot Zone- an area considered to be contaminated/or dangerous, due to a known or unknown agent.

Warm Zone- an uncontaminated zone into which contaminated victims may be moved. The Warm Zone may occur outside the Hospital Emergency Department as some contaminated victims may go directly to the hospital, by-passing the Emergency Medical Service (EMS), as was dramatically seen in the 1995 Tokyo subway incident where the Nerve agent Sarin was released, resulting in 12 deaths, with some 6,000 individuals, (the worried well), self-reporting to several hospitals, without apparent contamination of others.

Direct off-gassing from the lungs could be the mechanism for contamination in this scenario.

Cold Zone –this should be a completely uncontaminated zone unless patients have unknowingly contracted transmissible diseases e.g., small pox, pneumonic plague, viral hemorrhagic fevers.

If there is potential for exposure to blood of body fluid from a suspected or known contaminated patient, at a minimum, Level D precautions should be the rule.

Potential Risk associated with PPE: improper fit which may result in penetration.

Penetration – the process by which hazardous material may enter protective equipment via small cuts or breaks in the material.

Permeation – the process by which such materiel over time crosses protective barriers of the garment.

Degradation – the process by which structural elements of a product are decomposed by contact with chemical substances, leading to penetration and permeation.

Recontamination is possible for the user of PPE if proper protocol and training has not been adequate.

Droplet Precautions – designed to reduce the risk of droplet transmission of infection mucous particles larger than 5um (micrometer) in size. These may be generated by coughing, sneezing or talking by a person infected or a carrier, usually traveling 3 feet or less.

Airborne Precautions – designed to reduce the risk of airborne transmission of droplets 5um or smaller. There may remain suspended in the air or dust particles which may possibly be carried by air current longer distance. In these instances, special air handling and ventilation system are required.

Airborne precautions apply to patients known or suspected of being contagious with the potential for infecting others.

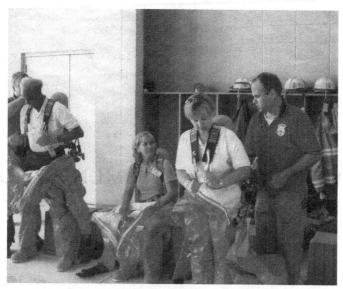

Figure 1. Author shown on the left putting on a Level A SCBA.

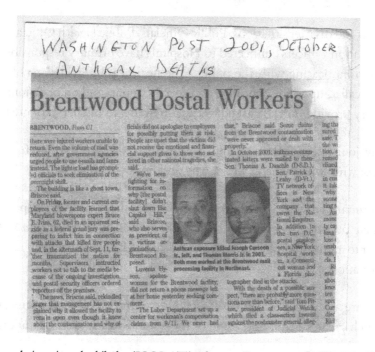

www.cdc/gov/nerdud/hihp/ISOLAT/airborne-Prec_excerpt/htm
www.cdc.gov/ncidod/hip/ISOLAT/droplet_prec_excerpt.htm
www.emedicine.com/emerg/TOPIC894.HTM

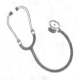

CHAPTER 3

HEALTHCARE RISK COMMUNICATIONS

"Strange how few, after all's said and done, the
things that are of the moment".

Edna St. Vincent Milla

In crisis and disaster situations, Public Officials, Public Health Officials[1] and Information Officers connected to Hospitals have primary responsibilities for communicating with the public. The healthcare provider may be the expert called upon for definitive and specific input, and on occasions, the primary provider may be asked to explain events to his/her patient(s).

Many journalists' often attempt to answer six key questions for their stories; who, what, where, when, why and how.

The primary provider would do well to try to do the same when responding to their patients, recognizing that at the outset of an event, and often well into its unfolding, they may have limited and possibly inaccurate information.

There are a number of sources which will address Risk Communication in much greater detail and some of these are listed. It is most important

---

[1] www.ATSdr.cdc.gov/HEC/Primer.html World Health Organization Outbreak, Communication Guideline, Communicating in a Crisis: Risk Communication Guidelines for Public Officials. U.S. Department of Health and Human Services Reprinted 2006, Rockville, MD.

that the provider be honest, open and frank. Be compassionate and clear when speaking.

Speak within your area of expertise, DO NOT SPECULATE!

If you do not know the answer(s) to the question(s) say you do not know but will try to get the correct information and get back to the individuals in a reasonable time. Remember you may be just as unaware of the immediate problem as are your patients, non-the-less they may look to you for information, guidance, and support. Try to have a definite time for follow up, even though you may not have all the information.

Always have a list of key contacts available with land lines, cell phones, e-mail, faxes of local Health Departments, and the CDC.

If you are on staff at various Hospitals, be aware of their emergency contact system for information; ideally becoming a part of a team or local Medical/Healthcare Reserve Corps. If there are Citizens Corps designated to helping in disasters, as is common is some areas, become familiar with this group.

Be sure to have an Emergency Operation Plan for your family and your office and be sure to practice your plan several times a year, in day-light and at night.

More about this in Chapter 11.

If you are called to act as an expert, work very closely with your Information Officer and with the Media, not FOR the Media, unless you are their employee.

Seven Cardinal Rules of Risk Communication have been put forth by Covella and Allen in 1998: [2]

1. Accept and involve the public as a partner.
2. Plan carefully and evaluate your efforts.
3. Listen to the publics' specific concerns.

4. Be honest, frank and open.
5. Work with other credible sources.
6. Meet the needs of the Media.
7. Speak clearly and with compassion.

These rules apply more appropriately to Public Health Officials and Information Officers who likely would be interacting with the Media and other officials; however, a well-informed healthcare provider with good risk communications skills, would offer a tremendous amount of comfort to their patients as events unfold in a major crisis.

For most healthcare providers a measure of crisis risk communications [2] may have been established; consider the Surgeon who has to tell the patient that the lump in her breast is a malignant cancer, or the parents of their teen-agers involved in an auto accident that they are dead, or the wife that her husband has had a heart attack, or the pediatrician who has to tell the parents that nothing more can be done for their five-year old child who has terminal Leukemia.

Of all the chapters in this book, the Author would implore the reader to become very familiar with risk communications as this is a major interaction in any walk of life between two or more individuals where trust and credibility should be paramount. [2]

As we write this chapter, having completed several others, we are mindful of the fact that as a country we are still awaiting another wave of the H_1N_1 pandemic influenza (swine flu to some). And although we as a country are deeply concerned about the economic downturn, we as healthcare providers should not forget the other flu pandemic, the H_5N_1 "bird flu" which is still circulating in the world, and for which there is inadequate vaccine.

And of course, Covid-19, about which much more will be discussed later.

The reader is referred to an article by Peter. M. Sandman, titled Pandemic Influenza Risk Communication: The Teachable Moment, posted 12-4-2004. [3]

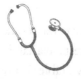

CHAPTER 4

BIOLOGICAL AGENTS

"Certain signs precede certain events".
Cicero

Following the Anthrax event of October 2001, a group of experts published the book, Bioterrorism: Guidelines for Medical and Public Health Management, JAMA Archives, Journal 2002.

The book should be in every healthcare provider's library, and frequently revisited. It describes multiple biological agents with the potential for causing considerable morbidity and mortality healthcare providers should be familiar with.

These agents have been grouped as Category A agents based on the following characteristics:

High Morbidity or Mortality.
Easily transmitted from person to person.
Lack of sufficient or available medicine.
Lack of sufficient or available treatment.
Capability of being infectious via an aerosol.
Potential to cause public panic and social disruption.
Potential for major public health impact.

Anthrax

Bacillus anthrax, gram positive bacteria, inhalational, cutaneous and gastrointestinal – diagnostic tests available, long term antibiotic therapy. Limited amounts of vaccine available; is not contagious.

Anthrax is an acute infectious disease caused by the Bacillus anthracis, a gram positive, "boxcar" or bamboo shaped rod. [1]

It is a spore forming, non-motile non hemolytic organism which can survive in the outside environment for years.

Anthrax most commonly occurs in wild and domestic animals, cattle, sheep, goats and antelopes. Prior to the events which followed after October 2001 with the deaths from anthrax, the author could find only 18 cases reported from sheep herders with Woolsorter's Disease.[5]

These individuals had the cutaneous form of the disease, seen in 95% of those affected. The infection may be from a cut or an abrasion in the skin from handling contaminated hides, leather products or hair, especially goat hair and a raised, itchy "bump" arises and within 1-2 days becomes a painless, popular, vesiclular ulcer, 1-3cm in diameter and finally a black necrotic eschar forms in 7-10 days. [2]

The other forms of anthrax infection and via the gastrointestinal tract and by inhalation. [GI]

Anthrax is not known to be transmitted from human to human. Eating undercooked meat from infected animals or by drinking water contaminated with the spores, which can lie dormant for decades [3] in an animal carcass, is a means of infection. It is an acute inflammation of GI tract with nausea, vomiting, lack of appetite, fever, and abdominal pain. The vomiting may be bloody followed by bloody diarrhea.

---

[2]   Roche KJ et al., NEJM 2001, P. 345-1611

[3]   Ken Alibek, Biohazard, Chapter 7, p.70-86, Random House Inc., 1991

Deaths from GI anthrax may occur in 25%-60% of cases improperly treated.

Cutaneous anthrax when treated with antibiotics is fatal in only about 1% of cases, however if untreated may result in a 20% fatality rate. [4] The most lethal form is Inhalation anthrax. The spores are inhaled as was the route of the cases at the United States Post Office in Washington DC in October 2001. [5] [see Washington Post article].

Symptoms of anthrax are categorized as "flu like" and occurs within 7 days of infection and may include a non-productive cough, chest discomfort, fatigue, shortness of breath and muscle aches. A fever with a temperature of 100 degrees F or higher may occur, possibly with chills or night sweats. Other symptoms are sore throat, difficulty swallowing, headaches and enlarged lymph nodes. The GI symptoms described may be noted with an incubation period of 2-43 days as seen in Russia. [3]

A lesion may occur on the face, arms or hands then progressing to the painless necrotic eschar noted. [2]

Inhalation anthrax which may result in meningitis and for shock may have a case of fatality rate of 55-75% even with supportive care and appropriate antibiotics. [7]

A distinguishing feature from the flu may be an absence of a runny nose in Inhalation anthrax. In any of the three forms the bacteria can spread to lymph nodes and abdominal pain and to the central nervous system producing Hemorrhagic meningitis which at autopsy may reveal the "Cardinals cap". [2]

Diagnostic methods include skin biopsy, for cutaneous anthrax, sputum testing, Chest X-Ray, and Computerized Tomography (CT) scan of the Chest, which will show a widened Mediastinum and Hilar nodes; also, blood tests for any form, endoscopy and stool samples and GI and spinal

---

[4]   www.bt.cdc.gov/documentsapp/anthrax/10312001/han51.asp

[5]   en.wikipedia.org/wiki/Woolsorter's _disease

top for suspected meningitis. Blood cultures should be drawn before antibiotics are started.[6]

CT should be non-contrast and bloody pleural effusion may be noted. Specific immuno-histochemical (IHC) and samples for polymerase chain reaction nasal swaps may be required.

Nasal swabs are not recommended by the CDC to determine if a person is infected with anthrax. A positive swap may indicate exposure and a negative swab does not indicate infection. Hospitals at Bio-safety levels 2, 3 and 4 are equipped to disguise anthrax.

Research since 2001 has identified Anthrax virulence factors as edema factor, lethal factor and protective antigen and the presence of a D-Glutamic Acid. The Anthrax toxins scheme Edema Factor and Protective Antigen= Edema Toxin, which causes edema in the skin. Lethal factor + Protective antigen = Lethal Toxin which kills most macrophages and animals. As noted earlier, Anthrax is not known to spread from human to human so there is no need to quarantine individuals suspected of being exposed to Anthrax or to immunize or treat contacts of persons infected.

Antibiotics for individuals post exposure include Cipro 500 mgm, p.o. q 12 hrs., Amoxicillin 500 mgm, p.o. q 8hrs. All should be given for at least 60 days. For inhalation anthrax Ciprofloxacin 400 mgm, IV q 12 hrs., or Doxycycline 100 mgm, IV q 12 hrs. Also, 1 or 2 of the following Clindamycin, Penicillin, Rifamin, Vancomycin, Imipenem and Chloramphenicol mgm, p.o. q 12 hrs, or Doxycycline 100 mgm, q 12 hrs., also for 60 days due to risk of inhalation anthrax.

[1] (www.BEPAST.org)

Infectious Disease Specialists should be involved in the management of all the organisms in Category A.

---

[6] Jerigan et al., Emerging Infectious Diseases, 2001; 7; p.933-944

For special populations such as the Military and those working in Research Laboratories with Anthrax, antimicrobial prophylaxis and use of Vaccines should be provided. [7],[9]

Post exposure vaccination is with 3 doses of the FDA licensed vaccine of 1, 2 and 4 weeks. For postal workers or those concerned or at risk from exposure, they showed follow "common sense" steps such as not opening suspicious mail, do not blow or sniff mail contents, avoid tearing or shredding mail products and wash hands after handling the products. Any suspicious packages or envelopes should be placed on a stable surface, alert others to avoid and notify security about suspicion immediately. Also thoroughly wash hands with soap and water. Some postal facilities have in place now the Anthrax Worker Safety Guidelines, recommended by the CDC and can be reviewed at reference.[8]

Some possible new therapies involve blocking of the Protective Antigen Core which prevents entrance of the lethal factor and Edema factor into host cells, also once a day Levofloxacin for treatment as post exposure prophylaxis and a nasal vaccine.

According to the Washington Post, in an article dated 8/5/2008, BIVIN borrowed from a Biology Lab freeze drying equipment, a Lyophilizer, that allows scientists to quickly convert these germ cultures into dry spores.

The Lyophilizer is commonly employed by laboratories as well as food processers to freeze a liquid broth of bacteria and quickly transform it into a dry solid without a thawing stage.

In June of 2008, the Justice Department agreed to pay Steven J. Hatfill, "a person of interest" in the case a $5.8 million settlement to forgo a privacy lawsuit. Another Washington Post article dated 8/4/2008 indicated that "the FBI made a genetic match between Anthrax spores from Bivin's lab and those used in the attack, including those taken from the victims' bodies".

---

[7]   MMWR, Novemeber 9, 2001

[8]   www.cdc.gov/mmwr/preview/mmwrhtme/mm5043a6.htm

It is important to keep in mind the role of Medical Examiners and Coroners (ME/Cs) in Disease Surveillance, collecting and reporting data, but also that those patients, with contagious Diseases, should not be embalmed. Standard precautions with blood products, aerosols, oscillating saws and contagious bags should also be used. Documentation should use standard forms, including Laboratory tests and stored in electronic databases.

There are Disaster Mortuary Operational Response Teams (DMORTS) which can protect the Scientists from airborne pathogens, respond to mass disasters from biological agents, support sampling for Class A and B organisms as well as store those records. [8]

Botulism

Gram positive bacillus may be food borne or aerosolized; diagnosis is by clinical suspicion, toxic assay serum.

Helpful clinical findings are the 4 D's, Diplopia, Dysarthria, Dysphonia and Dysphagia. There is no person-to-person spread by air.

According to Wikipedia, "Botulism [(B)] is a rare but potentially fatal illness, caused by the toxin produced by the bacterium Clostridium botulinum. Clinically there may be blurred vision, weakness of the arms, chest muscles and legs, also paralysis my occur. *

"In 1869, the German Physician John Muller, coined the term *botulism* from the Latin word *botulus*, meaning sausage". [1]

The botulism toxin was first described by Van Ermengen in 1897, after he investigated a food-borne outbreak in Ellezelles, Belgium. [2]

The classical [4 's of Dysphonia, Dysarthria, Dysphagia and Diplopia] may occur, with a 7th Nerve Palsy and Respiratory failure.

There are 4 types of Botulism, Foodborne [(Fb)], the most common, Infant, Inhalational and Wound. Wound botulism has been associated with street drugs, e.g., Black Tea heroin, seen in California. Foodborne is associated with improperly cooked foods. Infant botulism [Ib] has been associated with Honey, which can harbor the organisms, and should not be given to infants under 12 months old.

The Inhalational type may occur from inhaling the spores, which may be in the soil or water.

Botulism has occurred after Cosmetic use from the inappropriate strength of Botox administered. **

Diagnosis is made from clinical signs and symptoms in Infants and from testing the stool or enema specimen with the mouse bioassay. The organisms can be found with the enzyme-linked immunosorbent assays (ELISAs), and cultured from tissues.

There are 8 botulinum neuro-toxins, A, B, C (C1, C2), D, E, F, G which are antigenically and serologically distinct, but structurally similar. Human botulism is caused mainly by types, A, B, E and rarely F."

Treatment is currently with antitoxins, Ventilatory care and supportive measures. [Rx]

The paralysis usually last from 2 to 8 weeks, during which time Ventilatory and supportive measures are necessary.

In treated individuals the mortality rate is from 5% to 10%, but may be as high as 40% to 50% in untreated cases.

There is currently no Vaccine available, however, for Infants, BabyBig® provides a level of antitoxin antibody for 6 months.

[1] https://emergency.cdc.gov>agent>background.
[2] https://www.ncbi.nim.nih.gov>articles>PMC2856357.
[B] http://en.wikipedia.org>wiki>Botulism
[Fb] Schloss, D, Medical Intervention for Bioterrorism and Emerging Infections, Premier Ed., p 69-82, 2004
*Fact-sheets-Botulism

**Sobel J, (2005)" Botulism" Clinical Infectious Diseases, 41 (8): 1167-73.

(Rx) Medical Treatment for Botulism, https://www.ncbi.nim.nih.gov/pubmed/16452558.

(Ib)"Botulism Prognosis", https://www.news-medical-net/health/Botulism-prognosis.

Covid-19

The Coronavirus which was responsible for the Severe, Acute Respiratory Syndrome (SARS) in 2003 causing over 800 deaths and the Middle East Respiratory Syndrome (MERS) appears to be related to a number of deaths, 2000 and over 70,000 confirmed cases in 2020, allegedly originating in Wuhan China, but has spread to multiple countries as of this writing, according to Cable News Network (CNN).

On January 30 2020 WHO declared Covid-19 to be a Public Health Emergency of international concern. During this time there were ominous signs of the viral reproductive ratio called the "r-naught". This relates to how many infected individuals come from a single infected individual, or the contagiousness of the virus. It is generally agreed that an "r-naught" of less than 1 means that viral spread will fade over time.

According to the WHO in January 2020 16 Healthcare workers were infected with Covid-19. The virus appears to be a recombinant virus with its origin from a Bat. We remember that the origin of the virus for SARS is from the Civet Cat, and for MERS, from a Camel.

The first case of person to person (P2P) spread in the US was from a woman to her husband…she had recently traveled to China. Both were hospitalized and have since recovered.

As of February 13, 2020 there were 15 new cases in the US with no deaths. At that time the CDC warned against over reacting and that it was not necessary to wear face masks.

Information from the Food and Drug Administration (FDA) {permission *from FDA is not required for printing}* indicated the Incubation Period for the Disease is 2 to 14 days with a median of 4-5 days.

Clinical presentation is noted as:

Mild Illness-uncomplicated upper respiratory tract infection.
Moderate Pneumonia-upper respiratory infection without the need for Oxygen.
Severe Pneumonia-Dyspnea, shortness of breath, pO_2 < 93%, P/F <300
Critical-respiratory failure, septic shock, organ failure.

Other Covid-19 clinical findings include, Delirium, Hallucinations, Brain Fog, light sensitivity and excessive tearing, a rash, new loss of taste and smell, covid tongue and covid toes, nausea, vomiting and diarrhea, 14 days after contact with an infected individual.

Laboratory findings on Hospital admissions:

Lymphopenia 83%
Leucocytosis 34 %
C-reactive protein <_ 10 mg/L: 61%
Elevated Liver Function Tests, AST, ALT
Increased D-dimer is a strong predictor of mortality.

As of this writing, FDA recommended treatment for Covid-19 are likely forthcoming.

Drugs which are under consideration are:

Remdesivir Lipinavir/ritonavir
Hydroxychloroquine or Chloroquine (primary for Malaria, Lupus).
Zithromax

For Covid-19 refractory shock, low dose systemic corticosteroids are recommended.

In December 2021, Paxlovid (Nirmatelivar tablets, ritonavir tablets), became the first oral medication authorized by the FDA to treat covid in adults and children ages 12 years and older, at high risk for severe illness. *

*https://www.goodrix.com>condition>covid-19>fda-p.

Vaccines, as of 2/2/ 2021 from Moderna, Pfizer and Astra-Zeneca from the University of Oxford provide from 70 to 92 percent effectiveness, requiring either one or two injections.

Two such vaccines are COMIRNATY and Novavax.

Side effects and complications from the vaccines are still being tracked and recorded.

www.health.harvard.edu>blog>covid-19-vaccine-sa.

pO_2 should be at least 96% and supplemental O_2 is suggested for pO_2 of <92% and recommended for values < pO_2 of 90%.

With regards to intubation if required, Video guided Laryngoscopy is recommended rather than Direct Laryngoscopy.

Currents numbers of Global cases as of 2/21/2021 were total 11,921, 694 and 2,477,698 deaths.

"Globally, 772,166,517 confirmed cases, 6,981, 262 deaths and 3,595, 583, 125 vaccine doses were administered as of November 22, 2023" according to the WHO.[a]

In the United States, total cases as of 2/21/2021 were 28,752,348 and 510,930 deaths.

"In the United States, there were 103,436,829 confirmed cases and 1,138 confirmed deaths as of November 22, 2023". [b]

Clinical information related to the Covid-19 infection is often changing as more cases occur, more deaths will likely occur.

The author recommends updated information on covid-19 and other diseases discussed in this book be searched for at the CDC and Who.

https://www.cdc.gov/covid-19
https://www.cdc.gov/coronavirus/2019-ncov/hcp/therapeutic-options.html
https://www.cdc.gov/coronavirus/2019-ncov/hcp/
disposition-hosptalizd-patients-html
www.worldometers.info>coronavirus>country>US
a. htpps://www.who.int/Publishers>m>item
b. covid-19.who.int/regions/amro/countries/us.

Dengue

"Dengue and Dengue Hemorrhagic Fever (DHF), a mosquito borne infection, has become a major International health concern" according to the World Health Organization.

*htpp://www.who.int/mediacentive/factsheets/fs117/en/.

Dengue was first recognized in the 1950s during epidemics in the Philippines and Thailand.

"It is caused by one of four closely related, but antigenically distinct virus serotypes, Den-1, Den-2, Den-3 and Den-4 of the genus Flavivirus." **

**http://www.cdc.gov/ncidod/dvbid/dengue/.

"Infection with one of these serotypes provides immunity to that serotype for life, so persons living in a Dengue endemic area can have more than one infection in a life time". *

The female Aedes aegypti, a domestic day biting mosquito is the most common vector. The Aedes albopitcus can also infect humans.

They also transmit Yellow Fever, Chikungunya and Zika.

"In 1970 only Den-2 was present in the America's, although Den-3 may have been present in Colombia and Puerto Rico. In 1977, Den-1 was introduced, Den-4 in 1981, both causing major epidemics in Colombia and Puerto Rico". ** According to the CDC, "In 2005 Dengue is the most important mosquito borne viral disease infecting humans; its global distribution is comparable to Malaria, with an estimated 2.5 billion people living in areas at risk for epidemic transmission". **

Factors which appear to play a role in the global emergence are uncontrolled urbanization and population growth, substandard housing, inadequate water, sewer and waste management systems which increased the mosquito population and lack of effective mosquito control, and increased air plane travel." **

The WHO reported the following statistics in 2005.

"During the epidemic of Dengue, attack rates of 40-50 %, but may reach as high 80-90 %.

It is a severe flu-like illness which infects infants, young children and adults. The clinical features include a febrile syndrome, or the classic incapacitating disease with an abrupt onset of high fever, severe headache, pain behind the eyes, muscle and joint pains and rash.

Dengue Hemorrhagic Fever (DHF), a potential deadly complication, often with liver enlargement, fever 40 degrees C (104 F), febrile convulsions and circulatory failure. Symptoms usually last for 2-7 days.

The incubation period is 4 to 10 days.

There is no specific treatment for Dengue but intensive supportive care, including fluids, electrolytes and adequate nutrition has reduced the mortality rate to less than 1%. Without proper treatment, DHF case fatality rates exceed 20%". **

Data from the Dengue Surveillance Report ***indicates "that continued efforts of vector control, proper waste disposal and improved water storage practices should further control and reduce the spread of the disease".

In 2013 cases have occurred in Florida and in 2015, and an Outbreak of 181 cases were reported in Hawaii. **

*** https://www.denguesurveillance/dengue-andseveredengue.

Although the 4 serotypes of Dengue make it difficult to develop a vaccine for all 4, in 2015 and early 2016, the first Dengue vaccine, Dengvaxim (CYD-TDV) by Sanofi Pasteur is registered in several countries for use in individuals 9-45 years of age, living in endemic areas. ****

****https://enwikipedia.org/wiki/dengue_vaccine

Healthcare providers must always be cautious of any patients with unexplained viral illness and contact their local Department of Health and/or the CDC.

Glanders

Glanders was first described as a disease of horses by Hippocrates in 450 BC. [1]

Glanders (Farcy) is an infectious disease in humans caused by the bacterium Burkholderia mallei, described in 1949 by Walter Burkholder. [2]

Wilhelm Schultz and Friedrich Loffler, first isolated B. mallei in 1882 from the infected liver and spleen of an infected horse. [2a]

"The term is from Middle English glaundres or Old French glandres, both meaning 'glands". [3]

It primarily affects horses, donkeys, mules, goats, cats and dogs.

In 1940 it was noted to infect humans working in slaughter houses in contact with infected animals, and was used in the military as a biological weapon. [4]

Signs and symptoms may include fever, chills, sweating, muscle aches, excess tearing of the eyes and light sensitivity, ulcers and diarrhea, depending on the route of infection; the respiratory tract, nasal or oral mucosae or cuts and abrasions, 1 to 5 days after infection. Person-to-person infection may also be via bodily fluids. [5]

The septicemic form in humans has a high mortality rate, "case fatality rate of 95% in untreated cases and more than 50% in treated cases". [6]

With regards to the term 'farcy', it has been shown that "when nodules are in the lungs and other internal organs, the disease is glanders, and if nodules are mainly on the surface of the animal, the disease is known as farcy".[7]

Diagnosis is by finding the organism in saliva, blood, urine or skin lesions. [8]

The Mallein Test is a highly sensitive and specific and diagnostic htpps:// test for Glanders in horses. [8a]

There is no known vaccine. [9]

Therapy includes antibiotics, Sulfadiazine, Ciprofloxacin, Gentamycin and Tetracyclines. [10]

Infectious Disease consultation is strongly recommended.

[1] https://en.wikipedia.org.wiki>Glanders
[2] https://en.wikipedia.org>wiki>burkholderia_capacia
[3] htpps://en.wikipedai.org>wiki>Burkholderia_mallei.
[4] J Immunol., 1947; 56 (1) 7-96.
[5] https://www.ncbinim.nih.gov?articles/PMC3766238
[6] htpps://www.nj.gov>agriculture>divisions>diseases.
[7] https://www.gov.uk>guidance>glanders-and-farcy.
[8,8a] health.ny.gov/diseases/communicable/glanders/fact_sheet.
[9] https://www.uk>environment>food-and-Farmomg.
[10] Glanders/CDC www.cdc.gov>glanders.

Hanta Virus

Hanta Sin Nombre Virus. * (Sin Nombre-nameless, Wikipedia)

The Sin Nombre virus is a member of the genus Hantavirus which causes the Hantavirus Pulmonary Syndrome (HPS) or Hantavirus Cardiopulmonary Syndrome (HCPS). The mortality rate is between 40-50%. This is a severe acute respiratory illness, first reported in May 1993 in the Four Corners region of the United States, Utah, Colorado, Arizona and New Mexico (UCAN). In North America these viruses are carried by mice and rats, the deer mouse, the white-footed mouse, the rice rat and the cotton rat. The viruses are spread in the urine and droppings and breathed in or touched by humans. There have been some cases of human-to-human spread.

Clinical findings are a non-productive cough, fever, severe muscle aches, difficulty breathing and fatigue.

Other Hantaviruses such as the New York virus is found in the white-footed mouse.

"The Andes virus which causes the HCPS in Chile and Argentina, reportedly is the only Hantavirus which has been documented in human-to-human transmission."

** (J.P.Olano, D.H. Walker, in Vaccines for Biodefense and Emerging and Neglected Diseases, 2009).

Hantaviruses also cause Hemorrhagic Fever with Renal Syndrome (HFRS).

"Initial onset is marked by non-specific flu-like symptoms, albuminuria, and hemorrhagic findings include purpura, nasal bleeding, hematuria, hematemesis and Gastro-intestinal bleeding.

Diagnosis includes peripheral blood smears, chest x-rays and Serological Assays for serum IgG and/ or IgM.

Mortality is between 40 50 %.

IV Ribavirin has been shown to be effective during the early phase of HFRS illness". ***

No vaccines or specific treatment is generally available.

*http://www.cdc.gov/ncidod/diseases/hanta/hps/index.htm.
**https://www.sciencedirect.com/topics/medicine-and dentistry/sin-nombre-virus.
*** Omar Lupi, L. Klotz, Tropical dermatology, (2nd Edit.) 2017

Influenza

A patho-physiological process by which "infectious diseases or toxins are dispensed to cause disease is called dissemination". [1]

The same routes of entry pertain to natural spread of disease, inhalation ingestion and injection through the skin, and are also routes of entry from agents intentionally used as biological weapons.

"Biological agents are most likely delivered as aerosols via inhalation with resultant deposition within aerosols, which provides a direct pathway to the systemic circulation." (Figure1x.)

Droplets as large as 20 microns can infect the upper respiratory tract, however, these relatively large particles generally are filtered by natural anatomic and physiological processes with much smaller particles, ranging from 0.5 to 5 microns reaching the alveoli efficiently.

"Aerosol delivery systems tend to generate invisible clouds with droplets or particles between 0.5 and 10 microns in diameter which can remain suspended for long periods.

Smaller sized droplets are generally not efficiently retained by the human respiratory tract and are relatively unstable under ambient environmental conditions.

Infections via inhalation may induce respiratory disease at doses lower than generally associated with naturally acquired infections via the oral route with a subsequent illness which may differ from the natural internal and with a much shorter incubation period".

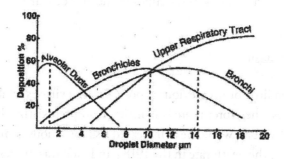

Figure 14. Droplet Size and Penetration of Respiratory Passages

(b) Aerosol delivery systems aim to generate invisible clouds with particles or droplets between 0.5 and 10 microns in diameter which can remain suspended for long periods. Smaller sized particles are not efficiently retained by the human respiratory tract and are relatively unstable under ambient environmental conditions. Infection by the respiratory route may induce disease at doses lower than those generally associated with naturally acquired infections by the oral route. The subsequent illness may differ from the natural pattern, and the incubation period may be much shorter.

(1) http://www.fas.org/nuke/guide/usa/doctrine/dod/Fm8-9/2ch1-htm.

Anthrax spores which can remain dormant for years, and with known techniques for developing aerosolized spores make it an interesting agent to use in biological warfare, and is noted here because of the "flu-like" symptoms which may occur early.

Clinical findings of patients exposed to bioterrorism agents may include "flu-like symptoms such as cough, fever, muscle aches, chills and fever. A pandemic flu and seasonal flu also are associated with similar findings but with these differences."

"Seasonal flu occurs annually, usually in the winter, in temperate climates and healthy adults are usually not at risk, with serious complications and deaths increased in the very young and elderly. There usually is an adequate supply of vaccines based on known flu strains available. The average death rate from pneumonia is approximately 36,000 per year and the social impact is modest with some school closings, and worldwide there is manageable impact on domestic and world economy."

A pandemic flu occurs rarely, three times in the 20th century as previously noted. [2]

[2] www.pandemicflu.gov.

"There had been little or no previous exposure to the viruses which caused these pandemics, therefore, there was little or no pre-existing immunity and healthy individuals would be at increased risk for serious complications and deaths. Note the death rate in the 1918 pandemic was highest in those aged 15-35 and health systems could be overwhelmed. Also, vaccines probably would not be available early in the pandemic and effective anti-virals could be in a limited supply."

"Recalling the estimated deaths in the 1918 USA, pandemic 500-600,000, the death rate could be quite high. Symptoms and complications could be severe causing a major impact on society with widespread restrictions or travel, closings of schools and businesses and large gatherings and generally wide spread social disruption." [3]

[3] www.pandemicflu.gov

The following information on influenza is taken from Wikipedia, 2/25/08 "the name influenza came from the Italian- influenza meaning 'influence' and latin -*influentia*". [4]

In humans, common symptoms are fever, sore throat, muscle pains, severe headache, coughing, weakness and general discomfort [1]. In more serious cases, pneumonia, which can be fatal in young children and the elderly, may occur.

Influenza spreads around the in seasonal epidemics and in the 20th century three pandemics have occurred, killing tens of millions of people. In the 1990s a novel avian strain H_5N_7 [7] appeared in Asia.

"The large death toll was caused by the high infection rate of up to 50% and the extreme severity of symptoms suspected to be caused by cytokine storms" [7a,7b].

As noted in the January 2005, Scientific America, [3] Jeffery Taubenberger and his group noted, "each of the three novel influenza strains that caused pandemics in the past 100 years belong to the Type A group of flu viruses, one of three main forms designated A, B and C. Type B and C infect humans only, but has never been known to cause pandemics. Type A infects a wide variety of animals including swine, poultry, humans and other mammals. Aquatic birds such as ducks serve as the natural reservoir for all the known sub types of influenza A, indicating that the virus resides the bird's guts without causing symptoms."

The Scientific America article noted that "On September 7th, 1918, at the height of World War I, a soldier at an Army training camp outside of Boston reported to sick call with a high fever. Doctors diagnosed him the next day when a dozen more soldiers were hospitalized with respiratory symptoms. Thirty-six new cases of this unknown illness appeared on the 16th, and by September 23rd, 12,604 cases had been reported in the camp of 45,000 soldiers. By the end of the outbreak one third of the camps population would be infected and nearly 800 would die. The soldiers who perished often developed a purplish skin color, many succumbing to suffocation. Many died in less than 48 hours after symptoms appeared and at autopsy their lungs were filled with fluid or blood, death now being ascribed to the cytokine storm noted above.

Most deaths were among young adults between ages 15 to 35 years old. Of note is the fact that antibiotics had not yet been discovered and most of the pandemic were due to pneumonia caused by appropriate bacteria. A subset of influenza victims died just days after the onset of symptoms due to a more severe viral pneumonia, caused by the flu itself with their lungs either massively hemorrhaging or filled with fluid."

This is one of the reasons vaccination against pneumonia with PCV15 or PCV20 is recommended for adults and the elderly.

A pediatrician should be involved with children.

This was based on "lung tissue obtained from individuals who had died in 1918 in an Inuit fishing village, now called Brevig Mission in the Seward

Peninsula of Alaska, preserved in permafrost, and from a lung specimen from a soldier who died in September 1918 at Fort Jackson, South Carolina. A soldier who also died in 1918 at Camp Upton, New York, and a woman of unknown age from the Brevig Mission, in collaboration with British colleagues with 1918 influenza victims from the Royal London Hospital, they were able to analyze and sequence the RNA virus responsible for the 1918 influenza. Wild avian strains can mutate over time or exchange genetic material with other influenza strains producing more viruses that are able to spread among naturally and domestic poultry. [4]

The virus's genetic material consists of eight separate RNA segments which reproduce the virus binds and then enters a living cell with new viral protein and copies of viral RNA being manufactured. If two different influenza virus strains` infect the same cell, their RNA sequences can mix freely producing progeny viruses that contain a combination of genes from both the original viruses. This re-assortment of viral genes is an important mechanism for generating diverse new strains.

Different circulating influenza A viruses are identified by referring to two signatures on their surfaces. One is hemagglutinin (HA) which has at least 15 known variants or subtypes. Another is neuraminidase (NA) which has 9 subtypes."

"The process of re-assortment occurring specifically in Influenza A is referred to as anti-genetic shift, [5] because it can affect humans as well as other mammals and birds. The natural mutation over time of known influenza strains and influenza B and C, which only infect human all though much less than A, is referred to as anti-genetic drift". [6]

"All influenza viruses experience some type of mutation which lessons the body's ability to respond with protective anti bodies, and therefore, vaccinations on a yearly basis are recommended." [6]

Since 1918, there have been a number of influenza viruses which have caused illnesses. As noted, by Taubenberger in the Scientific American article, "we must remember that the mechanisms by which the pandemic strain originate are not fully understood."

A review of clinical findings associated with inhalations of anthrax, plague, and tularemia reveal similar findings and depending up the scale of the bio-terrorist event the overall impact could be similar to those of a pandemic common symptoms of influenza may include "body aches, especially joints and throat, coughing and sneezing, extreme coldness and fever, fatigue, headache, irritated watering eyes, nasal congestion, dry eyes, skin, mouth, face, nose and throat and nausea and vomiting".[7]

Many of these findings are associated with biological and chemical agents which may be used by Terrorists.

On February 3rd, 2006 a new diagnostic test called the Influenza A/ H5C (Asian lineage) virus real-time reverse transcription polymerase chain reaction (RT- PCR) primer and probe set was available. The test provides preliminary results suspected in influenza samples within 4 hours whereas previous tests required 2-3 days.[8]

The Rapid Influenza Diagnostic tests are "immunoassays that can identify the presence of influenza A and B viral nucleoprotein antigens in respiratory specimens and provide results as either positive or negative".[9]

A swab of the throat is taken and sent to the laboratory and the results are available within 15-20 minutes. Some offices may have this capability.

Sensitivity ranges between 75-80% in Laboratories and in Physician offices between 50-70%

Specificity may be greater than 90%".

The Centers for Disease Control and Prevention (CDC) in the article "Influenza (FLU): Overview of Influenza Testing Methods," "last reviewed on 11/27/19 notes that "Positive and negative predictive values of an influenza virus test, depends upon the prevalence of circulating seasonal influenza viruses in the patient population compared to {a gold standard} comparison test (molecular assay or viral culture)."

[9] (See Guidance for Clinicians on the use of RT-PCR and Other Molecular Assays for Diagnosis of Influenza Virus Infections for more information CDC).

Treatment [10]

As noted, earlier because of the property of the influenza viruses to mutate vaccinations formulated for one year may be ineffective in the following year therefore, vaccinations must be given annually. The most common human vaccine is the trivalent influenza vaccine which contains material from two influenza A virus substrates and influenza B virus strains. [8]

There are four medications with antiviral activity against influenza viruses are commercially available in the United States. They are classified into two categories, the Adamantine derivatives and the Neuraminidase inhibitors. Although all four have been approved for use against the influenza viruses, they may not all be effective as resistance may develop.

The neuraminidase inhibitors are oseltamivir (Tamiflu) and Zanamivir, an orally inhaled powdered drug approved for chemoprophylaxis in persons aged 5 years and older and for treatment for influenza for ages 7 and older. Oseltamivir is approved for influenza treatment in person aged one year and older and for chemoprophylaxis in persons one year and older.

They block the activities of the emerging neuraminidase, reducing the number of viruses released from the infected cell. When used within 48 hours both drugs have been shown to be effective. The duration of each is 5 days.

The other medications are Amantadine and Ramantadine, drugs which are thought to interfere with influenza A virus and inhibits un-coating which inhibits virus replication resulting in decreased shedding.

Side effects of oseltamivir include nausea, vomiting; zanamivir with nausea, diarrhea, headaches. Some serious central nervous system (CNS) effects may occur. Zanamivir is generally not recommended for use in patients with underlying respiratory conditions. Antiviral resistance may occur.

Side effects of the adamantine drugs include gastrointestinal and CNS symptoms.

Before starting treatment with these antiviral agents, the healthcare provider should refer to the CDC information and recommendations.

As of October 1st, 2010, Codes 488.0 influenza, due to identified Asian influenza virus and 488.1, influenza due to identified novel H_1N_1 influenza virus were expanded in coding documents for purposes of third-party tracking and billing.

It is possible that these Codes will have changed by the time this Book is published.

A complete subdivision of these Codes can be found in the International Classification of Diseases (ICD-9-10).

3 www.scam.com

4 & 8 http://en.wikipedia.org/wiki/influenza

5. www.answers.com/topicantigenicshifts

6. www.answers.com/antigenics%20drift

7. www.hhs.gov/news/press2006/press/20060203.html

8. https://www.cancer>gov>dictionaries>cancer-drugs>def

9 CDC Guidance for Clinicians on the use of RT-PCR and Other Molecular Assays for Diagnosis of Influenza Virus Infection for more information.

10.http://www.cdc.gov/flu/professionals/antivi-ralback.htm

Respiratory Syncycial Virus (RSV)

RSV is now one of the most common respiratory infections involving the very young and the elderly.

According to the CDC, "Respiratory Syncytial Virus (RSV) * is a virus that usually causes mild, cold- symptoms from which most recover in one or two weeks; however, in infants and older adults, it can cause serious illness.

It is the most common cause of pneumonia and bronchiolitis in children younger than one year of life.

Symptoms include runny nose, coughing, sneezing, wheezing, fever and decrease of appetite.

Older adults with underlying diseases may require hospitalization and mechanical ventilation.

Transmission is by viral droplets from coughing or sneezing, close contact, surface contacts or door knobs, and is usually contagious in 3 to 8 days.

There is no specific treatment, and current therapy includes control of fever and pain, fluids and rest."

*https://www.cdc.gov/rsv/

The Washington Post Newspaper reports on page A4, May 8, 2023, "The first vaccine to prevent the respiratory disease caused by RSV was approved this week by U.S. regulators for use in adults 60 and older. Depending on the season, 60,000 to 120,000 older adults are hospitalized in the United States with RSV each year, and according to the CDC 6,000 to 10,000 die.

The new vaccine, called Arexvy, developed by the pharmaceutical GSK, contains a harmless version of a protein found on the outside of the virus.

In a clinical trial with nearly 25,000 participants, Arexvy was shown to be 83% effective in preventing lower respiratory tract disease caused by RSV in older adults. It was 94% effective against severe disease.

Other vaccines are in the making, such as Abrysvo, and in June, 2023, experts who advise the CDC on vaccines are expected to meet to make recommendations on how approved RSV vaccines should be integrated into the public health care".

Legionnaires` Disease [1] (Pontiac Fever, * Legionnellosis)

This a severe type of pneumonia, caused by the Legionella bacteria.

It is not generally passed from person-to-person, acquired as an aerosolized respiratory infection, inhaled from contaminated water, or less frequently, from swallowed contaminated water.

It was named in 1976 following an outbreak in Philadelphia, Pennsylvania at an American Legion`s meeting. [1]

Symptoms are flu-like, including fever, headache, cough, shortness of breath and muscle aches. [2]

There are "specific diagnostic tests, indicated if patients have failed outpatient antibiotic treatment for community acquired pneumonia, immunocompromised patients with pneumonia and those with pneumonia in a setting of a Legionella disease out-break, and testing for health-care associated Legionnaires disease.

At risk factors include age over 50, chronic lung disease, diabetes, renal failure disease and immune system disorder or medications.

Best practice diagnostic tests are sputa, ideally before antibiotics are given, and a urinary antigen test concurrently.

The urinary antigen detects Legionella pneumophilia serogroup1, the most common cause of the disease, although there are some 60 different species.

The preferred agents for treatment include the Macrolides and the respiratory fluroquinolones…management should be directed by Infectious Disease Specialists.

The disease is fatal in about 10% of cases overall and in 25% of healthcare associated disease; however, most people exposed to the bacteria do not become ill.

Public health officials must be notified of cases in a facility." [3]

1. https://www.cdc.gov>legionella
*Pontiac Fever-https://www.cdc.gov>travel-related-infctious-diseases

In 1908, several healthcare workers were diagnosed with legionnaires disease in Pontiac, Michigan.

2. htpps://www.cdc.gov/legionella/fastfacts.html.
3. www.who.int>news-room>fact-sheets.

Leprosy [1]

Leprosy was often noted in the Bible over 2000 years ago. [2]

It is "A contagious disease that affects the skin, mucous membranes and nerves, causing discoloration and lumps on the skin, and in severe cases, disfigurement and deformities.

Common signs and symptoms include runny nose, dry, reddish skin, muscle weakness loss of sensation in the fingers and toes, atrophy of the testes and impotence." [1]

With the frequency of international travel, it should be included in the Differential diagnoses of skin diseases.

The cause of the disease was identified by Gerhard Armauer Hansen, a physician in Norway, as Mycobacterium leprae in1873. [2,4]

There are about 120 to 250 cases diagnosed in the USA each year. [3]

Transmission is primarily via the Upper Respiratory Tract. It is not transmitted via sex, nor passed via the placenta at birth. [5]

Mycobacterium lepromatosis is another name noted by the CDC.

Diagnosis is made by finding the acid-fast leprae Bacilli in skin smears and by polymerase chain reaction (PCR) methods. [6,7]

Guideline for diagnosis and treatment, prevention of Leprosy has been established by the WHO, and the standard treatment, as of 1981, is multi-drug therapy MDT), using 3 drugs, rifampicin, dapsone and clofazimine. [8]

---

[1] https://en.wikipedia.org/wiki/Leprosy.

[1a] The New American Bible, Confraternity of Christian Doctrine, Washington, DC, 1977, Mark 1:40-42.

[2] Jour., of Dermatol, 39 (2):121-129, Feb., 2012, Current Status of Leprosy, Suzuki, K, Ishii, N, et.al.

[3] CNN.com/2019/02/21/health/leprosy-cases-study-index-html.

[4] International Textbook of Leprosy, Pathogenesis and Pathology of Leprosy, 11 Feb., 2016, Retrieved 22 July 2019.5

[5] cdc.gov/leprosy/transmission.com

[6] WHO.int/leprosy/diagnosis/en.

[7] PCR-based Techniques for Leprosy diagnosis in the Clinic; Neglected Tropical Diseases, 8(4): e2655.doi10_/journal. pnid.000265.pmg 3983108pmid24722358.

[8] Guidelines for the diagnosis, treatment and prevention of Leprosy, WHO, Regional Off., E Asia, 2018_p xiii, hdl:10665/274127, isbn-978-9022-6383.

Lyme Disease

Lyme disease is the most commonly reported vector-borne disease in the US, mainly in Maryland, Virginia and the North East. It is caused by the Bacteriun Borrelia burgdorferi, transmitted most commonly by vector-borne ticks such as Ixodes scapularis or Ixodes dammini.

It may present in 3 stages, localized, disseminated or persistent.

Initially, it may present as an expanding red-ring (Bulls Eye) rash, Erythema migrans, with headache, fever, malaise and arthralgias. *

Diagnosis is aided my Enzyme Immuno-assay (EIA) or Immunofluorescent Antibody Assays (IFA) tests.

Treatment is with antibiotics, often Doxycycline; however, an Infectious Disease Specialist should be involved in management.

*NIAID History of Lyme Disease:

https//www.niaid.nih/gov-diseases-conditions/Lyme-disease.

As of April 2019, the World Health Organization (WHO) listed 8 diseases likely to cause severe epidemics in the near future. [1]

Crimean-Congo Hemorrhagic Fever, Ebola, Marburg Fever, Lassa Fever, Middle East Respiratory Syndrome, (MERS), Severe, Acute Respiratory Syndrome (SARS), Nipah Valley and Rift Valley Fever.

Highly pathogenic emerging coronaviruses that affect humans such as CoV(covid-19) is becoming a major problem.

This was discussed earlier and much more information will likely be available by the time this Book is published, one such entity being *'long covid'.*

Long covid is considered to be a noun *, with post covid -19 symptoms including extreme fatigue, muscle weakness, breathlessness. The CDC defines it as occurring when one who was initially infected and has not been able to return to their usual state of health in 4 or more weeks. **

An Infectious Disease Specialist should be involved with management of these patients.

Lassa Fever has a death rate of 15-20%. Eighty percent of those infected may be asymptomatic but does require contact and respiratory isolation, as does Marburg and Ebola.

Nipah Valley and Rift Valley affects animals and humans.

Chikungunya [2] is a viral disease transmitted by mosquitoes, the Aedes albopictus and Aedes aegypti, which causes fever and severe joint pain and swelling, headache, conjunctivitis and a rash in 50% of individuals diagnosed. Symptoms are similar to those with Dengue Fever and Zika Fever.

Diagnosis includes clinical findings, laboratory findings are mainly a decreased lymphocyte count, reflecting the viremia, and confirmed by viral isolation, serological studies and RT-FCR.

As of 2017 there was no approved vaccine or treatment.

*https://www.apta.org>news
**www.everydayheath.com/coronavirus-what is long-covid.
[1]   diseases-likely-to-cause-major-epidemics. [2]https://en.wikipedia.org/wiki/chikungunya.

Nipah was first recognized in March, 1999 named after the town of Nipah in Malaysia in an outbreak of encephalitis, inflammation of the brain and respiratory illness in men.

The virus belongs to the paramyxovirus family which includes measles, mumps and Hendra viruses. A total of 211 persons, including 59 deaths were reported from 2001 -2005 due to Nipah virus [3]

Men in Singapore working in abattoirs *(a slaughter house for animals)*, and around pigs were also infected. Over 900 pigs were culled in Malaysia and abattoirs were closed and a ban on transporting pigs.

Onset appears to begin in 3-14 days with a fever, headache, flu-like respiratory symptoms and signs which may progress to drowsiness and coma within 24 hours. During the outbreak in 198-1999, 405 of those with serious nervous disease hospitalized died.

Human-to-human spread has not been shown but fruit bats may be the reservoir that leads to infection of pigs, which can infect humans, cats and dogs via close contacts.

The drug Ribavirin has been shown to be effective against the viruses in vitro however, no vaccine or specific treatment is available at this time.

Hendra virus disease, from the family para-myxoviridae also, was first isolated in 1994 in a suburb of Brisbane Australia, according to the CDC Fact Sheet. Between 1994 and 1995 two outbreaks occurred with 15 horses and 3 humans, one of whom survived. [4]

Clinically there was an influenza-like illness (ILI) with fever, myalgia, cough, shortness of breath and neurologic illness with meningitis. Human infection occurs by close contact with body fluids from infected horses. No air borne transmission has been documented, nor human to human spread.

The "Flying fox" bat appears to be the reservoir, also for the Nipah virus.

There is no known vaccine or antiviral drug treatment. [3] [3]https://www.cdc.gov.vhf/nipha/pdf/factsheet.pdf

[4]Medlindia.net/patientinfo/nipah-virus-niv-or-hendra-virus.htm.

Diseases caused by Parasites, except to note Plasmodium which causes Malaria, and those described in Food Borne diseases.

One important reference is noted. *

* CDC, about Parasites. https://www.cdc.gov/Parasites/about_html.

Plague

Yersinia pestis, gram negative bacterium, fever, cough, hemoptysis and air borne with person-to- person spread; surgical masks for patients and healthcare workers. Described as the Black Death in the past, and is associated with flea infected rats. May present with a rash or enlarged inguinal lymph nodes termed *bubo inflammation* treatment must be started early, 6-24 hours before final diagnosis known. Sputa, blood cultures and gram stains are indicated.

Mortality may be as high as 50% if early antibiotic therapy is not started. Plague is an infectious disease caused by Yersinia partis. It is a gram negative, non-motile, non-spore forming, pleomorphic bacillus, named by Alexandre Yersin and Shimbasa- Buro Kittaso during the Hong Kong Plague epidemic in 1894. [1]

[1] Perry, RD, et.al, Yerterina pestis-etiological agent of plague. Clin. Microbiol., Rev 19997;10:35-66.

The first documented pandemic is recorded in the, 1 Samuel 24:15. [2]

2 The New American Bible, 1977, Confraternity of Christine Doctrine, Washington, DC, 1 Samuel 24:15.

The Black Death or threat pestilence occurred in 1346 in 14th century with the death toll exceeding 42 million. [3]

In nature the hosts for the bacillus includes wild rodents, squirrels and prairie dogs, also domestic pets e.g., dogs and cats. Fleas are the major vectors for spreading the disease. The Oriental Rat flea Xenopsylla cheposis has been the vector most commonly associated with natural transmission with the black or brown Rat being the host reservoir. The human flea, Pulex irritans was implicated during the Black Death. [4]

When the disease remains confined to the wild animal population i.e., enzootic, the flea- rodent cycle is maintained.

If the disease is more widely spread among the animal reservoir, i.e., epizootic, there may be an animal die-off, and the fleas seek other hosts, including humans. This factor becomes important in management with contrast of the fleas being most important before animal control.

This is clinically important because it takes only 1 to 10 organisms to transmit the plague bacillus.

Humans may contract either by flea bites, which is the most common route and causes Bubonic Plague which is the most common manifestation in man, with over 75% of naturally occurring cases. [5] The other primary clinical forms are septicemic and pneumonic with meningitis and pharyngitis as possible complications.

When a human is bitten by an infected flea, an ulcer or pustule develops at the site and after an incubation period of 1-8 days lymph node enlargement occurs proceeded by fever, chills, which may become effectively tender. With early and appropriate intravenous antibiotic therapy, incision and drainage is generally not required.

Septicemic plaque may present with fever, chills, abdominal pain, diarrhea hypotension and multi-organ failure. Petechia and purpura may occur along with disseminated intravascular coagulation (DIC) and acral necrosis of the fingers and toes which was noted with the Black Death. Mortality may reach 50%. [6]

Primary pneumonic plague may be acquired via inhalation of the organism or from on aerosolized form, which is the most likely form a terrorist would use. Secondary pneumonic plague and the primary form maybe acquired via hematogenous spread from Bubonic or septicemic plague. The incubation period in from 1-6 days. Primary pneumonic plague is transmittable from human to human and animals to human, therefore, contact and respiratory isolation is necessary. Those infected as well as healthcare workers and caregiver must have protective surgical masks.

Diagnosis is by culture of sputa, blood and aspirates of enlarged lymph nodes. The aspirate should consist of a 10 mL springs containing sterile saline infected into the enlarged node. Cerebrospinal fluid and scrapings from skin lesions can also be cultured. Patients with pulmonary plague may develop cough, shortened of breath, chest pain and hemoptysis and respiratory failure.

When sending material to the laboratory suspicious for plague, the laboratory workers must be notified, and biosafety level and safety conditions must be in place.

Pneumonic plague may be confused with other fulminant forms of pneumonia. Also, other conditions may produce buboes such as Tularemia,

Catch-Scratch disease, Chancroid and Chlamydia, Lymphogranuloma venereum and Tuberculosis.

Chest X-Rays may show additional infections, consolidation, and cavitating disease, none of which is pathognomonic for pneumonic plague. [7]

Gram negative rods with bipolar staining with Giemsa, Wright, or Wayson, staining with a "safety pin" appearance may be seen, but can also be seen in Escherichia coli; Klebsiella and Pasteurella. Direct Fluorescent Antibody and Polymerase Chain Reaction (PCR) available at the CDC.

The mortality rates have been reported at 50% or higher if treatment has not started before 24 hours. Effective antibiotic therapy has included Doxycycline, Ciprofloxin and Gentamicin, as well as Streptomycin and Chloramphenicol. Pneumonic plague may be confused with other pneumonia and forms of pneumonia illness, the health care workers should consult with an appropriate specialist, Infectious Disease in this case, for proper management as with any serious or uncommon infectious illness. Keep in mind the effects of the illness on special populations i.e., children, pregnant females, the elderly, and those confined, e.g., Nursing Homes and Prisons.

Further, since Plague is one of the Category A agents with the potential for use as a bioweapon, the appropriate healthcare and law enforcement agencies should be contacted urgently, as it is critical to differentiate a naturally occurring outbreak from a possible bioterrorism event.

The World Health Organization (WHO) has reported that an estimated release of 50 kg of Yersina pestis over a city with a population of 5 million, resulted in 150,000 clinical cases and up to 36,000 deaths. In this hypothetical scenario, it reported, some 80,000 to 100,000 would require hospitalization and isolation.

"An exercise involving the release of Yersinea pestis into the Performing Arts Center in Denver, Colorado", is reported by Michael Roy, Physician Guide to Terrorist Attack, Chapter 6, plague, p.89, 2004 Hanona Press. [9]

There were "3,700 cases of pneumonia plague deaths and also of particularly grave concern, were the potential problems in leadership and decision making as well as the confusion regarding distribution of resources" that were highlighted by the TOPOFF exercise, as noted by Inglesby and O'Toole. [10]

[3] Asken, F, Cecil JC, "The Influence od Disease Upon European History", Mil Med 1983: 148-441.

[4] McGovern, TW, Friedlander, AM, Plague IN: Sidell et.al., Textbook of Military Med, Aspects of Chem and Bio Warfare, Borden Institute, Wash., DC, 1977, p479-502.

5 Palmer, D, Plague In: Gorbach, Bartlett, JG, et.al., Inf. Dis, 2nd Ed., WB Saunders, Phila., Penn., pp1568-1575

6 Hull, HF, Montes, JM, et.al., "Septicemic Plague in New Mexico", J. Infect., Disease 1987:113-118.

7 Aslofrom, DJ, Mann, JM, "Radiographic Manifestations of Plague in New Mexico",1975-1980, Radiology 1981; 139:561-565.

[8] WHO, Health Aspects of Chem and Biol Weapons, WHO, 1970, pp107-109.

[9] Michael Roy, Physician Guide to Terrorist Attack, Chapter 6, Plague, p.89, 2004 Hanona Press.

[10] Inglesby, T, O'Toole, T, "A Plague on your city: observations from TOPOFF: Clin infect Dis., 2001;32:436-445.

Rocky Mountain Spotted Fever (RMSF)

RMSF is the most common tick-borne Disease caused by the Bacterium

Rickettsia rickettsii in the US, transmitted by one of several ticks, the American dog tick and the Rocky Mountain wood tick. *

Symptoms may include high fever, headaches, nausea, vomiting, a rash on the wrists and light sensitivity.

Diagnoses includes skin biopsies, blood tests and the *gold standard* IFA serological Test. **

Antibiotics, including Doxycycline are used for treatment.

** Bratton RL., et al,Tick Borne Disease, Am. Fam. Physicians, 2005:71(12);2323-2330.

Small Pox

Variola major, a DNA virus requires contact and respiratory isolation needs fit tested N-95, N-100 or PAPR masks, also negative pressure room. Diagnosis is based on clinical suspicion, a rash on the face, oral cavity, hands. Vaccination with a bifurgated needle, up to 3-4 days is effective in decreasing morbidity and mortality; the main differentials are Chicken Pox, Measles and drug reaction. The Investigational New Drug (IND) Cidofovir offered under FDA approval may be effective. In June, 2021, the drug Brincidofovir (Tembeka) (CM-X001) was approved by the FDA for treatment of Small pox and Tecovirimat (ST-246), for which the FDA indicated the treatment outweighs the risks. *

There is no antibiotic therapy.

*cdc.gov/smallpox/clinicians/treatment.html.

The center for Disease Control and Prevention (CDC) describes Small pox as "an acute, contagious and sometimes fatal disease caused by the DNA variola virus – symptoms may include a fever > 101 F and one or more of the following; headache, backache, chills, malaise, fatigue, vomiting, and abdominal pain".

There are two forms of small pox, Variola Major and Variola Minor".

According to a guide to diagnosis and management of Category A bioterrorism agents [BE PAST] by Daniel Lucey et. al, [BP]

"The incubation period is 1-17 days and includes a Febrile Prodrome period, 1-4 days before the onset of a rash; classic lesions, deep seated firm, round vesicles or pustules which may have umbilication or confluence; then all the lesions are in the same stage of development initially or the face, mouth, palms, sole arms the trunk. The scab falls off the fulfilled particularly in about 21 days".

Most individuals who contract small pox recover but the death rate may be about 30% in individuals with Variola major ** and 1% Variola minor (Alastrim). Some individuals will have permanent scars and some may be blind. The disease is contagious, spread by person to person contact with infected individuals either as an airborne agent or by other bodily fluid; or from contaminated bedding or clothing.

Small pox was deemed eradicated in the works 1977 and in 1972 in the United States. In 1980 the World Health Organization (WHO) recommended that all countries stop vaccinating for small pox. Given these data and from why own review of the alternative, many physicians in this country have never had personal experience with patients with Small pox. Given this lack of clinical review and the "flu like" symptoms as described the prodromal period above, when the health care provider is presented with a patient with an unknown rash, they need to consider immediately contacting the local Department of Health about his or her concerns. A definite diagnosis of Small pox can be made by positive cultures, electron microscopy and polymerase chain rection (PCR).

When an individual is suspected of being infected with Small pox [as having been exposed to an infected individual] that individual should be vaccinated. The vaccinia virus which cannot cause Small pox is the live virus used for vaccination. Healthcare providers may/should be vaccinated unless they are in a group for which vaccination or is not recommended.

Individuals with Eczema or Atopic Dermatitis, allergies to any of the ingredients in the vaccine, pregnancy, or plans to become pregnant within one month of becoming pregnant and those under 12 months of age, should not be vaccinated. (Close discussion with an Infectious Disease Specialist is required).

In any event a discussion with one's Primary Care Physician or Ob-Gyn Physician should be had in the event there is the possibility of close contact with an infected individual.

Vaccination is thought to provide full protection for at least three years.

The CDC* notes "If there is a non-reaction or an equivocal reaction, vaccination must be repeated.

Between 14 and 52 individuals per 1 million (0.02%) vaccinated for the first time, experience potentially life-threatening reactions.

Individuals who have contracted small pox and have survived are generally thought to be immune to the disease. Vaccination is carried out by using a bifurcated needle and trained individuals should perform the vaccination.

The CDC has specific information for vaccination. There is no one specific proven treatment for Small pox and timely vaccination is currently the most appropriate method of managing the disease. The antiviral drug Cidofovir to date has been used under an FDA Investigational New Drug (IND) Protocol for treatment and serious vaccine reactions. According to the CDC vaccination within 3-4 days of exposure to the small pox virus could significantly reduce the severity of the disease. There are some significant complications which can occur from the vaccine such as Eczema vaccinatum, Generalized Vaccinia, Progressive Vaccina, Erythema Multiforme and rarely, Vaccinia Keratitis".

[BP] www.BEPAST.org.
*www.bt.cdc.gov/training/smallpoxvaccine/reactions.
**https://www.who.int>tems>vaccinestandardization.

If any healthcare provider sees or suspects and individual is infected with or has been exposed to one with Small pox, or has been exposed, the local Department of Public Health should be contacted immediately.

Tuberculosis

Tuberculosis (TB)[1] is an infectious disease, usually spread by Mycobacterium tuberculosis, 1a discovered by Robert Koch, a German Bacteriologist in March of 1882.[2]

He also discovered the causative agents for Anthrax and Cholera. It may occur in one of three stages, Active Disease, Exposure or as a Latent event.

The name tuberculosis was first coined in 1832.[1a]

According to the Center for Disease Control (CDC),[3] over 13million individuals are estimated to be living with Latent Disease and is found in 60 jurisdictions, states, cities, and Regions in the United States.[3] Without intervention, 10% will develop Active Disease.[3] World-wide, it is the 13th leading cause of death and second leading cause of death after Covid-19 above HIV.AIDS).[4]

Symptoms include productive, prolonged cough, hemoptysis, chest pain, fever, night sweats, loss of appetite and weight loss and anemia.

Due to the extreme pallor of the skin from the anemia*, Tb has been called "The Great White Plague and the White Death". **

It was also referred to as consumption in the past.

Spread is by droplet nuclei when infected individuals cough, sneeze, speaks or sings, from person to person.

The most common sites of TB are the lungs, pleura, central nervous system, lymphatics, bones joints, the genito-urinary system and miliary spread.[1]

The evaluation of individuals begins with a medical history, physical examination, chest x-ray a/or chest CT, sputa exam and skin testing, using the Purified Protein Derivative (PPD), the Mantoux test, describer in 1912 by Charles Mantoux (French).[5]

The Quantiferon Gold Plus TB blood test is considered the "gold standard" test for TB.[8]

Active Bacilli in the sputum and chest x-ray are need to see if active disease in present.

Intradermal injection of 0.1 milliliter (ml) of the derivative should be performed, producing a wheal of 6-10 millimeter (mm), and the induration should be "read" by a trained healthcare worker in 48 to 72 hours, and recorded in millimeters.

A measurement of 5-10 mm is classified as "Positive".

In some individuals a reading of 15 mm may be noted as "positive" but may not reflect Active Disease, thus the need for distinguishing a "False Positive from a False negative" reading. This may arise in instances where an individual may have been given the Bacillus of Calmette and Gueran (BCG),[6] however the test is not used in the USA.

"Also, the issues with 'anergy', (a condition in which the body fails to react to an antigen), as in a recent infection in the age group 6 months, or with overwhelming disease.

Anergy testing is no longer routinely recommended, including individuals who are HIV positive". [7]

Risk factors which increase TB infection include, substance abuse, diabetes mellitus, silicosis, head and neck cancers, end stage renal disease and HIV,[4] which is the strongest.

Factors contributing to the rise in Active Tb in the USA include a decline in the United States Public Health structure, increased immigration from countries with high TB rates and increase in HIV/AIDs.[4]

In 1943, Selman Waksmas discovered a compound called streptomycin which was given to a patient with TB in 1949, resulting in a cure.[9]

Later other drugs were developed for treating TB which were Ethambutol, Isoniazid, Pyrazinamide and Rifamycin.

The methodology, specific therapy and duration of therapy must be made in consultation with Public Health officials.

Healthcare workers are at increased risk for infection and active disease, so strict reporting of infected individuals and isolation measures mut be in place, as well as accurate outpatient follow when therapy is completed.

Multidrug TB (MDR-TB) resistance has developed and is a major concern to public health officials.[10] and is a Category C Bioterrorism agent.[11]

1https://www.cdc.gov>tb>publications>preventions.

1ahttps://www.cdc.gov>tb>worldtbday-history.

2https://www.cdc.gov>mmwr>preview>mmwehtml.

3cdc.gov/tb/statistics/default.htm.

4https://www.who.int>digital>tb-disewase-burden.

5https://en.wikipedia.org.wikiMantoux_test

6https://www.ncbi.nim.nih.gov>booksNBK538185.

7American Family Physician, 2000; 62 (7)

8https://nmshealth.com>quantiferon-gold-plus-compound

9https://en.wikipedia.org/wiki/Selman-Waksman

10https://en.wikipedia.org>wiki/History_of_tuberculosis

11https://emergency.cdc.gov>agent>agentlist-category

Viral Hemorrhagic Fevers (VHF)

These viruses are in Category A and include, among others, Ebola and Marburg, Filoviruses and Lassa and Machupo, Arena Viruses; all are transmittable from person to person. [BP]

Healthcare providers need fit-tested N-95 or N-100 masks or powered air purifying respirators.

Symptoms include high fever, red eyes, rash. Infection with the Lassa virus may cause pharyngitis and abdominal pain. Diagnosis is by clinical suspicion, specific viral isolation tests.

Currently a vaccine is in development and treatment is largely supportive.

In addition to Small pox, caused by the variola virus, a number of other viruses can be used as potential bio-weapons. There are four groups which ae the Filoviruses, Ebola, and Marburg, the Arena viruses, Lassa Fever and the New World Hemorrhagic Fever, Bunya viruses, Rift Valley Fever and Hanta Virus and the Flavivi Virus and Omsk Hemorrhagic Fevers are representative. ([1,2])

Usually, these infections are transmitted to humans by mosquitoes, ticks, or infected rodents. Routes of infection are by inhalation of aerosolized excreta or urine. direct physical contact with infected syringes among healthcare workers, sexual transmission and in cases of Rift Valley Fever, ingestion of contaminated raw milk. Clinical findings include flu-like symptoms, fever, headache, myalgia, abdominal pain, hemorrhagic conjunctivitis, pharyngitis, nausea, and diarrhea.

The Ebola and Marburg viruses can be found in blood and sweat.

The common vector for these two diseases appears to be the Fruit Bat.

The mortality rate of Ebola Hemorrhagic Fever is 50-90%, Marburg 23-70% and Lassa Fever 15-20%. Diagnosis of the Viral Hemorrhagic Fever requires the use of Bio-safety Level 4 Laboratories using the techniques of virus isolation ELISA and PCR as presented in Chapter 6.

Local Health Departments should work closely with the CDC in Atlanta or with the US Army Medical Research Institution of Infectious Diseases (USAMRID) in Frederick, Maryland, if these diseases are suspected. [1]

These agents can be delivered in an aerosolized form and potentially could be used as a bio-weapons. In addition to notifying the local Health Departments, an Infectious Disease Consultation should be obtained, and the suspected infected individual(s) should be isolated All Healthcare personnel must use appropriate PPE and exercise strict barrier protective measures.

There is a licensed vaccine for Yellow Fever and investigational vaccines are being developed.

There were no antidotes or vaccines for the Filoviruses Marburg and Lassa Fever; there is however for Ebola in 2018. [1]

Ebola

Ebola occurred as an outbreak in the Sudan in 1976, with 284 cases and confirmed 151 deaths (284/151). In Zaire (The New Democratic Republic of the Congo) there was a fatality rate of 88%, (318/280). Incubation is between 2 -21 days, with the usual onset of symptoms in 5-7 days. Deaths are usually between 6- 16 days. In non -fatal cases, individuals may have fever for several days and improve around day 6.

A possible reservoir is the fruit bat or Primates, such as the Ape or Monkeys.

The virus is thought to enter the human host via the mucous membranes or abrasions on the skin. During the outbreak in West Africa between 2014-2016, the majority of cases occurred between ages 15 to 44 years.

The dead should not be embalmed but buried in a sealed casket.

Without vaccination the fatality rate is between 50-90 percent, however as of 2022, survival rate has been shown to be 29.2%*

A vaccine, rVS-ZEBOV (Ervebo), was approved by the Food and Drug Administration (FDA) in December, 2019. It appears to be fully effective after 10 days.

(e)https://www.cdc.gov>vhf>ebola>clinical>vaccine.

As of the end of 2019 greater than 100,000 individuals have been vaccinated.

Treatment** must be coordinated the CDC, and 2 drugs have been approved for treatment, Inmazeb a mixture of three monoclonal antibodies and Ansuvimab-zykl, (Ebanga), a monoclonal antibody given by injection.

At this time, there is no cure for Ebola.

*https://www.cdc.gov>vhf>ebols>prevention
**https://www.webmed.com>ebola-fever-virus-infection.
CDC.gov/vhf/ebola/index.html.
Who.int/news-room/fact-sheets/detail/ebola-virus-disease.
en.wikipedia.org/wiki/ebola-virus-disease.
National Institutes of Health, https://www.nih.gov
Feldmann H, Geisbeert, TW, Ebola hemorrhagic fever, Lancet. 2011; 377:849-862.
Mahanty S, Bray M, Pathogenesis...Lancet Infect Dis, 204;4:487-498
WHO Response Team, Ebola virus...N Engl J Med.2014;371:1481-1495.
Baize S, et.al., Emergence...N Eng J Med., 2014;371:1418-1425.

Ribavarin has been used in cases of Lassa Fever and Rift Valley Fever. Rift Valley Fever found in Africa, South Arabia and Yemen is spread by mosquitoes which can infect livestock. When humans are infected, they may have retro-orbital pain, photophobia, retinitis and jaundice. There is no known person to person transmission of Rift Valley Fever, however, there could be a mosquito to human to livestock cycle.

Alpha Inferon has been suggested for treating Rift Valley Fever.

[BP] www.BEPAST.com.
[1,2] Henderson, DA, O'Toole, Bioterrorism, Guidelines for medical and public health management, JAMA Archives Journal 2002, p191-220. www.amapress.com product number 05445502.

Marburg Virus

In the early part of this year, 2023, the Washington Post News Paper reported an uptick in Outbreaks of the Marburg Viral Hemorrhagic Fever, one of the Category A Diseases.

"The name Marburg (meaning Frontier Fortress", was first used in 1130 when the site belonged to landgraves of Thuingia. The city's early history is associated with St. Elizabeth of Hungary who arrived there in 1228, and spent the remaining three years of her life there doing charitable work". [1]

"Marburg virus was first recognized in 1967, at the Philipps University in Marburg, Germany, when Outbreaks of hemorrhagic fever occurred simultaneously in laboratories in Marburg and Frankfort Germany, and in Belgrade, Yugoslavia [now Serbia]". [2]

The disease was named Marburg virus, after the West German town of Marburg van der Lahn, where most of the human infections and deaths occurred, where the laboratory workers were handling samples from African green monkeys imported from Uganda". [3]

In an article reported in the Washington Post News Paper, on February 15, 2023, entitled "The Marburg Outbreak: Deadly virus is highly infectious. The virus has surfaced for the first time in Equatorial Guinea, causing at least 9 deaths. It is a highly infectious viral hemorrhagic fever, spawned by the animal-borne RNA virus of the same Filoviridae family as the Ebola virus. [4, BP]

According to the WHO, symptoms can begin 'abruptly, including high fever, chills, malaise, sever head aches as well as abdominal pain, nausea, diarrhea and jaundice. Around day 5 a non-itchy rash may occur on the chest, stomach or back. In fatal cases, death usually occurs 8 or 9 days after the infection starts.

Fatality rates have ranged between 24% and 88%.

The largest Outbreak occurred in Angola in 2005, where more than 350 people were killed, according to a report from its Health Ministry.

According to the CDC, the virus is not known to be native in other continents such as North America.

There are no known Vaccines or approved anti-viral treatment". [4]

On March 24, 2023, The Washington Post reports "Outbreaks of Marburg virus have killed a total of 12 people in Equatorial, Guinea and Tanzania. The virus is not known to be air-borne, but can be transmitted by exposure to bodily fluids such as saliva, blood and urine; it can also be passed on by contact with contaminated materials and surfaces such as tables and door knobs.

A report from the Inter-govern-mental Panel on Climate Change noted that scientists think that Climate Change is driving and exacerbating outbreaks of the disease". [5]

[1].britannica.com/place/Marbug_Germany
[2.] https://pubmed.ncb.nim.nih>gov>
[3.] htpps://www.sciencedirect.com>medicine-and-denistry.
[4.] The Washington Post, February 15, 2023
[5].The Washington Post, March 24, 2022

Tularemia

Francisella tularensis, gram negative bacterium. No person to person spread by air, may present as febrile illness, pharyngitis bronchitis, pneumonitis hilar lymphadenitis, shock. It may appear as an ulcer on the extremities, an ulceroglandular type, typhoidal or in a meningeal form. The most common reservoir is the rabbit, and as few as 1 to10, organisms, up to 50, is all that is required to infect. Clinical suspicious is important. A chest x-ray may show broncho-pneumonia, pleural effusion or adenopathy. The lab will use gram stain of blood or sputa, a PCR, or Direct Fluorescent Antibody. Prescription antibiotics for 12-14 days are required.

Tularemia sometimes called Rabbit Fever, is caused by Francisella tularemia a small non motile aerobic gram negative cocobacillum which is non spore forming and can survive for weeks low temperatures in water, moist soil, hay and decaying animal corpses [9]. It is one of the most infectious

---

[9]   O Saslaw 5, Prior F., et al., tularemia vaccine study, arch Int Med: 1961, 107: pp. 121-146.

pathogen bacteria known requiring as few as 1 to 10 organisms to cause disease, even up to 50 organisms.[10]

A number of small animals such as moles, mice, rodents and squirrels are reserved and vectors are ticks, flies and mosquitos.

The rabbit in the most common reservoir.

Human infection can occur from noncultivation from tick bites, handling infected animals or animal products, or ingestion and inhalation of the organism.

Francisella tularensis occurs in two major subspecies, type A [11] and type B [12] based on virulence, biochemical reactions and epidemiological features. There are 6 major clinical symptoms of Tularemia [13].

Ulceroglandular disease is the most common form. Clinical findings depend upon the route of inoculation and the virulence of the organisms, type A or B [14].

The incubation period is from days 2-10 days with individuals presenting with fever, cough and flu-like symptoms and lymphadenopathy and lymphadenitis in the ulceroglandular form. Chest X-Rays may show plural effusion, pneumonia, hilar lymphadenopathy or a miliary pattern and typical infiltrates similar to tuberculosis.

There is no known person to prior spread. Oropharymgeal tularemia may occur from ingesting injections organisms and present with pharyngitis, abdominal pain, vomiting and diarrhea. The oculoglandular form may

---

[10]   Hopla, CE, The ecology of Tularemia, ADV Vet Sci Comp med. 1974; 18: 25-53

[11]   Tellison, wL, tularemia in North America, Missoula University of Montana 1974: 1-276

[12]   Garyova D. First isolation of Francisella tularensis in Europe. Eoi and Epidemics 1998; 14: 797-782

[13]   Schlorsberg D., Medical interventions for terrorism and emerging inspection, premier edit, 2004, p.44-51.

[14]   Evans, M.E., Mcgee ZA. Tularemia: a 30-year experience with 88 cases. Medicine 1985, 61: 251-269.

occur from direct inoculation of the eye from an aerosol or accidental auto inoculation or as a splash in laboratory workers.

A primary pneumonic involvement may occur from inhalation of the organisms, possibly among farmers sheering sheep, or among laboratory workers (5 p.44-51). Typhoidal tularemia is the most fatal form and resembles typhoid fever from hematogenous spread of the organism to a particular organ. There is no person-to-person transmission. The highest incidence of naturally occurring disease in the summer months when tick-borne and mosquito transmission occurs and again in the winter during hunting season.

The deer fly (chryson dixalis) and tick (ambyroma americanium) are common vectors. Tularemia could result from an airborne aerosolized route or contamination of the water supply. Scholorberg (5 p.45) reports that "water borne outbreaks of tularemia were documented during World War II when large number of Russian Troops were sickness from water contamination following disruption of urban sanitation".

The World Health Organization (WHO) has estimated that release of 50 kg of F. tularensis and inhaled over a city of 5 million could result in 250,000 illness and 19,000 deaths. A high degree of clinical suspicious is needed to help identify the first high risk patient with tularemia. A cluster of previously healthy individuals with a severe pneumonia or recent travel to an area known to be endemic for Tularemia. [15]

Outbreaks in Martha's Vineyard in1978 and 2000 were noted. [16]

Cultures should be taken before antibiotics are started. Because of the high risk of aerosolization and this identification, cultures should be only be attempted in RSL-3 laboratories and laboratory worker should be alerted to "rule out tularemia, according to Dr. Dan Lucey, reporting from the DC Hospitalization's Association, Infectious Disease Committee on Oct. 2, 2005". [7]

---

[15]   Lucey, D. et al., DCHA, DIC Committee, Oct.2, 2005

The two organisms most often misidentified as Francisella tularemia are Actinobacillus actinomycetemcointious and Hemophilus influenza. Other diagnostic tools include direct fluorescent antibody (DFA, ELISA and PCR). [8]

Special media containing cysteine or ceptine for growth are required to isolate the organisms.

Chest X-Ray and Cat Scan of the chest may show bronchopneumonia, hilar adenopathy or plural effusion.

Treatment should include any of the following antibiotics Streptomycin, Gentamicin, Doxycycline or Ciprofloxin for Tularemia, if thought to have been intentionally released.

Publications by DT, Henderson DA [16] describes Tularemia as a biological weapon, JAMA 2001; 285: 2764-2773.

As previously noted, management of Tularemia should be done with consultation from Infection Disease Specialists and coordinated with the local health departments and the CDC.[17]

The case fatality for Type A West is 0% compared to 7% with Type B, when treated appropriately, and type A East, 14%.

[17] Wildpro.tuycross200.org/5/00dis/bacterial/disease_tularemia/disease_ tularemia_litreps/DFA-Direct Fluorscent Antibody PCR-Polymerase chain reaction ELISA-enzyme-linked immunosorbent-assay.

West Nile Virus (WNV)

West Nile Virus is a seasonal epidemic illness, often seen in North America, which usually begins in the summer, continuing into the Fall.

According to the World Health Organization (WHO), "The WNV as first discovered in a febrile adult woman in the West Nile district of Uganda in 1937".

(WHO) https://www.who.int>news-room>fact-sheets>detail.

The symptoms include fever, headache, body aches, skin rash on the body and trunk and swollen lymph nodes, usually between 3 and 14 days after the bite.

According to the CDC, about 80% of individuals will be asymptomatic. (cdc) http://www.cdc.gov/ncidod/dvbid/wstnile/wnv_factsheet.htm.

The first cases in the Americas were noted in New Yok City in 1999. (Clinical Infectious Diseases [CID] 2000; 30:413-418). These were a cluster of 5 patients in August 1999 with fever, confusion, weakness, then paralysis.

Diagnosis was made after the exam of dead birds at the Bronx Zoo and human autopsy revealed the West Nile Virus.

Spread is by the bite of an infected mosquito, usually the Culex pipiens or Culex tarsalis species.

Methods of diagnosis include Antibody and nucleic acid tests, IgM enzyme immunoassay (EIA), IgG antibody, Nucleic acid-amplification and Virus isolation tests.

There is no specific treatment or vaccine at this time for WNV.

The main differential is with the Saint Louis Equine virus.

The WNV may be spread by blood transfusions, breast feeding, and from mother to fetus during pregnancy. It is not spread from casual contact.

The mortality rate, expressed as the case-fatality is "2% of patients aged,50 years old; 6% aged 50-60 and 21% aged _> 70 . (cf) (cf) https://www.cdc.gov/mmwr>volumes.

Zika (CDC)

The name Zika comes from the Zika Forest in Uganda, where the virus was first isolated from a Rhesus monkey in 1947. The first human case was noted in 1952.

The disease is spread by the bite of an infected mosquito, the Aedes aegypti or the Aegis albopictus.

Symptoms are "flu-like", which include fever, headache, a rash, red eyes, and muscle and joint pain. Many are asymptomatic.

Zika can be spread from a pregnant mother to the fetus, and by sex.

It has been known to trigger the Guillain-Barre Syndrome and in the pregnant female, it has been shown to cause *microcephaly. (m)*

To date, no cases have been documented to have spread via blood transfusions; however, in Brazil, Platelet transmission has been documented.

(m)who.int/news-room/fact-sheets/detail/Zika_virus.

The disease was first noted in Puerta Rica in 2016, then Florida. (zk)

(zk) https://www.statists.com>topics>zika-virus-disease.

There is no specific treatment.

In April 2017, subunit and inactivated vaccines have been entered in clinical trials. (ct)[See discussion on Vaccines, Chapter 11].

(cdc) cdc.gov/zika/index.html.
(cdc)https://www.cdc.zika>about>overview.
(ct) Fernandez, E., Diamond, MS., (April 2017) Vaccination on strategies against Zika virus, Current Opinion in Virology 23:59-67.

Category B Agents

Foodborne Pathogens which could be used as bioweapons include Escherichia coli, Shigella, Salmonella and Staphylococcus aureus, the latter having been implemented with the topic shock syndrome associated with tampons, and later with the systemic inflammatory response syndrome (SIRS).

Waterborne pathogens include Vibrio cholerae which is reported to be infecting a large number of individuals in Haiti and Cryptosporidium which infected more than 400,000 individuals from the drinking water in Milwaukee, Wisconsin in 1993.

An excellent summary of the above waterborne pathogen is presented by Schlorsberg. 1

A summary of an overview of Entero- Hemorrhagic Escherichia Coli (EHEC) is also reported by WHO on December 2001 follows. (1,2)

Escherichia coli is a bacterium community found in the intestinal tract of humans and warm-blooded animals. Whereas most strains are harmless, E. coli 0157; H-7 has been involved in a number of outbreaks in humans transmitted primarily from eating contaminated food products such as raw or undercooked means, milk, vegetables, sprouts and lettuce. Symptoms may include fever, abdominal pain, vomiting and diarrhea which may become bloody. The inhibitor period varied from 3-8 days with the young and the elderly more prone to life threatening illness such as the Hemolytic Uremic Syndrome (HUS).

The syndrome includes acute Renal Failure, Hemolytic Anemia and Thrombocytopenia with a Case Fatality rate of 3-5%.

HUS is the most common cause of acute renal failure in young children. Neurological complications such as seizure, stroke and coma.

Most individuals recover in about 10 days.

Waterborne transmission from contaminated drinking eater and recreational water has been reported. The organism has been found to survive for months in manure and water troughs. (2)

Of late, a number of recent outbreaks shave been associated with contaminated sprouts and lettuce, and contact with domestic and wild animals and feces.

Oral-fecal transmission has been noted with person-to-person contact. There is an asymptomatic carrier state where individuals are capable of infecting others, but show no clinical indication of illness themselves.

Prevention of infection requires diligence from farm to pork, including production, processing manufacturing and preparation of food products in household and community facilities.

The role of industry in prevention of infection requires safe clean hygiene slaughtering practice as well as education and training for individuals handling food chains. (2)

The WHO overview notes "the only effective method of eliminating EHEC from food is to introduce a bactericidal treatment, such as heating, 'cook thoroughly so that the center of the food reaches at least 70 C' pasteurization) or radiation". (2

Fruits and vegetables should be washed with fruits peeled if possible.

At risk individuals such as the very young and elderly showed avoid consumption of raw products and undercooked products. The EHEC produce toxins known as verotoxins, or Shiga-like toxin because of their similarity to the toxin produced by Shigella dysenteria.

Treatment requires fluids and electrolyte replacement and according to WHO, "antibiotics are not a part of the treatment for EHEC disease and may possibly increase the risk of subsequent HUS".

These agents are moderately easy to disseminate, have moderate morbidity and low mortality rates. They also require specific aspects of the Center for Disease Prevention and Control (CDC) diagnostic capability and enhanced disease surveillance. Some of the more common agents are:

Brucellosis – several Brucella species, and Cholera.
Epsilon toxic – Clostridium perfringens.
Food safety threats –Escherichia coli – 0157:H7. Shigella, Salmonella.
Legionnaires Disease (Legionnellosis, Pontiac Fever) {Discussed earlier}
Psittacosis – Chlamydia psittaci.
Q fever – Coxiella burnetii.
Ricin toxicity – Ricinus communis from caster beans.
Staphylococcal enterotoxin B.
Typus fever –Rickettsia prowasakii.
Viral encephalitis – Eastern, Western, Equine.
Water safety threats – Vibrio cholera, cryptosporidian parvan.

Cholera

Cholera is an infection of the small intestine caused by the bacterium vibrio cholera. Following the earthquake in Haiti in 2010, where 200,000-316,000 [1] were estimated killed, cholera has become epidemic. The Haitian Health Ministry reported the numbers of dead to be 1,024 with hospitalization over 16,700 as of November 16th, 2010. [2] Transmission is primarily due to fecal contamination of food and water due to poor sanitary conditions. The primary symptoms are vomiting, severe and painless diarrhea with losses up to 10-20 liters a day. [2]

The diarrhea also known as rice water diarrhea can contaminate water used by others [2] according to Wikipedia (11/25/2010).

Cholera affects 3-5 million people and causes 100,000 – 130,000 deaths worldwide as of 2010. Cholera has been found in only two other animal populations such as shellfish and plankton. [2]

Additionally, it is reported that Tchaikovsky and his mother died of Cholera and former President James K. Polk died from an outbreak in North America in the mid-1800s.

John Snow (1813-1858) demonstrated that human sewage contamination was the most probable disease vector in two epidemics in London in 1854 [3] and was the first reportable disease [1] in the USA due to its effect on health.

In 1885 Robert Koch identified the Vibria Cholera bacillius and later it would be classified as serogroup O1 and serogroup 0139. In Cholera epidemics the most common organism found in the Vibria Cholera O1. A clinical diagnosis should be made with a good history and physical exam in epidemic situations and treatment started before definitive laboratory confirmation. Stool specimen and/or a swap specimen should be sent to the appropriate reference labs in coordination with local health departments.

A rapid dip-stick test is now available. [4]

Developed countries with advanced water treatment and sanitation practices, Cholera can be prevented. Chlorination and boiling water are inexpensive and effective measure as well as effective sanitation for sewage. The earthquake in Haiti in January 2010 followed by the hurricane with diminished sanitation measures [2] and the close being quarter of the inhabitance were all causes in the outbreak that occurred. [1]

Proper disposal and treatment of sewage, with sanitization of possible contaminated materials using solar water disinfection, ultraviolet light sterilization and thorough hand washing are effective.

Multiple Cholera pandemics have occurred since the first was reported 1816-1826. Between 1865 and 1917, an estimated 2 million deaths in Russia occurred. [5]

The last outbreak in the United States was in 1910-1911 in New York City [6] where 11 people died including a health worker. Another report indicated at least 58 deaths.[7]

Generally, Cholera can be successfully managed with oral rehydration using rice-based solutions. [4]

In some instances, up to 10% of a person's body weight in fluids may need to be replaced. Ringers Lactate is the preferred solution II and electrolytes, especially potassium must [3] be covered. Antibiotics should be given after the correct organism is identified.

Overall management should be done in consultation with Infectious Disease Specialists.

When diagnosed and properly treated early the mortality rate is reported at less than 1%. When treatment is delayed or with under treatment, mortality rate may rise to 50-60%. [2]

[1] MSNBC 16, Nov., 2010. 1,034; Official Cholera death toll in Haiti passed 1,000. en.wikipedia.org/2010-Earthquake-Haiti.

[2] Sack, DA, Sack, RR, et.al., Cholera, Lancet363 (9404):223-233, Jan., 2004.

[2,3] Dr. John Snow, The Mode of Communication of Cholera, London, 1855.

[4] Sack, DA, Sack, RR, et.al., Getting serious about Cholera N. Eng. J. of Med. 355 (7): 649-651, Aug., 2006.

[5] The Early American Review: httpp://www.earlyamerican/com/review/2000_fall/1832_cholera_part 1.html.

[6] Cholera kills boy. New York Times, July 18, 1911

[7] Markel, H, "Knocking out the Cholera", Cholera, Class and Quarantine in NYC,1892, Bull. Hist Med 1955; 69:420-457.

Q-Fever

The "Q" stands for "Query" and was applied at a time when the cause was unknown.

It was first recognized as a Human Illness in Australia in 1935 and in the United States (US) in 1940.

It is an obligate intracellular bacterium, apparently named after Herald Rea Cox by C. B. Phillips in 1948. *

About "five out of ten individuals infected by Coxiella burnetii will get infected, usually 2-3 weeks after exposure with flu-like symptoms". Clinical findings may include chills and fever, sweats, chest and stomach pain, headache, non –productive cough and weight loss. Symptoms may be mild to severe and some individuals may be asymptomatic. Females who are infected are at increased risk for miscarriage, still birth or low weight infants. Some individuals may develop Chronic Q Fever, months or years later after being infected and develop Endocarditis.

Human infection occurs from inhaling dust from contaminated urine, feces and from eating unpasteurized milk products.

Animals such as sheep, goats or cattle are infected from eating contaminated products from infected animals.

Diagnosis depends on the Clinical History of association with certain animals and Laboratory tests.

As of 2017 there were 153 acute cases and 40 chronic cases reported.

Treatment includes Doxycycline and Hydroxychloroquine for several months.

*.en.wikipedia.org/wiki/Coxiellaburnitii#History_and_Naming cdc.gov/qfever/stats/index.html.

Ricin

A classic case is that of a 49-year-old male, who suddenly developed leg pain from an apparently accidental injury to his leg from an umbrella while awaiting a bus. Within 15-28 hours he developed nausea, vomiting and fever and he was admitted to the hospital. Within 36 hours increasing fever, tachycardia and lymph node swelling developed and at 48 hours, hypertension and shock developed, despite medical attempts at resuscitation.

By 72 hours anemia had developed, as had hematemesis and cardiac failure, and by hour 84 he was pronounced dead; presumed cause of death, Septic Shock.

At autopsy a "pellet" removed from his leg turned out to be Ricin and follow up investigations would reveal that Gregor Markov, a Belgian Journalist was assassinated by injection from an umbrella. *

Ricin is a compound from the castor bean plant (Ricinnus communis) a commercial source of castor oil. Patho-physiologically, it acts as a cellular toxin which blocks protein synthesis via modification of ribosomal 28s subunit.

Routes of exposure are inhalation, ingestion and parenterally.

The LD_{50} for Ricin is 0.05mg/kg, about the size of the head of a pin. There are no known antidotes for ricin toxicity, and only supportive measures for management are available.

On October 22, 2003 Ricin was found in a US Postal facility in the District of Columbia, later found to have originated from Greenville, South Carolina and the author, at that time the Medical Director for the Emergency Medical Health Service Administration (EMHSA) of the District of Columbia Department of Health called a midnight teleconference with various Public Health Professionals from the DC, Maryland and Virginia to discuss the event.

There were no health care events associated with the agent, nor with any other incidents in DC with which the author would be involved.

*https://en.wikipedia.org>wiki: Gregor Markov.

Food Borne Disease

According to the CDC, "Contaminated food results in 600 million cases of Foodborne Disease and 420, 000 thousand cases world-wide every year.

In the United States of America (USA), Noro virus is the most common cause of illness from food and water".

The Norovirus is considered to be the most common cause of acute gastroenteritis, diarrhea and vomiting (nv). The Centers for disease Control and Prevention (CDC) estimates that noroviruses are responsible for more than half of all food-borne disease outbreaks each year. The norovirus was originally called the Norwalk virus since the first case was confirmed in the town of Norwalk, Ohio. There are many types of noroviruses and exposure to one type may not protect from other types. (nv)

Norovirus is not related to the flu.

Infection comes from eating or drinking contaminated food, touching materials infected by the virus, then touching the nose, eyes or mouth (nv). The virus thrives in close quarters, cruise ships, day-care centers and nursing homes. Young children and the elderly are highly susceptible, due to weakened immune systems.

Clinical findings include vomiting, more often in children, and watery diarrhea, more in adults and stomach cramps. Other findings may be low grade fever, chills, headache muscle aches and fatigue.

Noroviruses cannot be treated with antibiotics and there are no antiviral drugs available at this time. (rx).

Treatment for Noro virus illness is rest and fluids as this illness usually resolves itself in a few days.

In the USA, 48 million people get sick, 128,000 thousand are hospitalized and 3,000 thousand people die from foodborne illness each year.

Foodborne Disease may be caused by any of the following 6 organisms;

Noro virus, Salmonella, Clostridium perfringens, Campylobacter, E. coli and Listeria, and several parasites, Trichanella spiralis (Trichanosis) and Taenia solium (Pork Tape worms), and Toxoplasmosis gondi, in undercooked meat. *

*https://www.mayoclinic.org>syc-20356249.

Some of the causes of Foodborne Disease are infected persons, contaminated raw food, inadequate heating and cooking, use of leftovers and cross contamination".

Fungal Diseases

These are some of the largest categories of diseases healthcare providers will encounter and ideally should be managed by Infectious Disease Specialists.

The WHO lists the most common fungal infections, with the most dangerous being "the critical group Aspergillus fumigatus, Candida albicans, Candida auris and Cryptococcus neoformans. Cryptococcus and Aspergillus are both invasive fungi and can infect the lungs". *

Aflatoxins.

"These are a family of toxins produced by certain fungi found on crops such as peanuts, maize corn, cotton seed and tree nuts. The main fungi that produce Aflatoxins are Aspergillus flavus and Aspergillus parasiticus.

People are exposed to Aflatoxins by eating contaminated plant products, such as peanuts or meat contaminated by animals that ate the contaminated flood". [1]

Farmers and agricultural works may be exposed by inhaling dust generated during the processing and handling contaminated products. [2]

"Exposure to Aflatoxins is associated with an increased risk of Liver Cancer.

Exposure can be reduced by buying only commercial brands of approved by the Food and Drug Administration, and discarding discolored or moldy looking nuts.

As of January 2020, no outbreak of human illness has been reported in the United States." [af]

The above information noted is as per the statement from the National Cancer Institute, "Unless otherwise indicated, all text within the National Cancer Institute (NCI) products is free of copyright and may be used without permission.

Credit the National Cancer Institute as the source". *

[af] https://www.cancer.gov/about-cancer/causes- prevention/risk/substances/aflatoxins
*WHOnpr.org/sections/goatsandsoda/2022…WHO- release-list-of-Threating-fungi.

From an article entitled Testing the Antidotal Efficiency in the Treatment of Aflatoxin Poisoning by Gradelet, S, Astorg, P, Suschetet, M., et al., the following information is noted.

"The effects of intoxication with aflatoxins were experimentally determined by oral administration to mice.

By comparing the essential elements of mycotoxins related to human pathology, they tried to estimate the protective role of a medicine usually administered as an antidote, Vitamin A.

It was administered in different quantities before, during and after the ingestion of foods with aflatoxins.

Early hepatic and late renal lesions were noted pathologically.

Administration of high doses of Vitamin A partially protected the animals and reduced the mortality to less than half.

They recommended that prophylactic or therapeutic carotenoids be administered to individuals exposed to aflatoxins". [va]

va https://limk.springer.com/chapter/10.1007/978-94-011- 4641-8_19

Correcting these causes eliminates or decreases chances for contracting these diseases.

[1] https://www.cdc.gov>foodborneburdens.
[2] https://opentex.ca>food>chapter>cause-of-foodborne.

Whenever any of these diseases are suspected, an Infectious Disease Consultation should be obtained for proper management.

Aspergillosis, is a fungal or mold infection, caused by Aspergillus fumigatus, usually involving the respiratory system, but may infect other body parts, as a fungus ball, and can be invasive. [1]

Symptoms include fever chills, cough, hemoptysis, chest or joint pain and skin lesions.

Diagnosis includes clinical findings, chest x-ray, Cat Scan (CT) of the chest, sputa and blood tests and skin biopsy. [1.]

Treatment my include corticosteroids, Amphotericin-B, or other anti-fungal agents. Invasive Aspergillosis may require hospitalization.

If a fungal ball is in a cavity, e.g., the sinuses, surgery may be indicated.

[1].https://www.cdc.gov/fungal.diseases/asperigollos/definition.html.
[2].www.mayoclinic.org>asperigillosis>SYC-20369619.

"Candidiasis is an opportunistic fungal, yeast, infection, most commonly caused by Candida albicans (C. albicans), which normally lives on the skin, in the mouth, the throat, the gut and in the vagina, usually causing no clinical problems".[1]

"An overgrowth of C. albicans in the mouth may cause Thrush, appearing as white raised bumps. Vaginal infection may present with itching or a white, cottage-cheese-like discharge, and an Invasive form may involve blood, bone, brain and the heart.

Symptoms may include itching, blisters, a reddish skin rash or as septic shock (Candidemia).

Normally, fungal infections are not contagious however, C. albicans has the potential to spread to different hosts, e.g., in immunocompromised hosts.

Diagnosis includes clinical evaluation, history of overuse of antibiotics, and cultures of the infected part. Endoscopy with appropriate cultures of the gut may be indicated." [2]

"More than 90% of patients with HIV present with Candidiasis.

Other predisposing factors include TB, vitamin A, B6 and Iron deficiency, smoking, poor dental hygiene and infancy and old age.

Treatment include anti-fungal creams in1,3 and 7-day courses.

Medications include amphotericin-B, Clotrimazole, Miconazole and Nystatin". [3]

If Dental Stomatitis is suspected or present, Dental Consultation is indicated, as well as Infectious Disease Consultation, depending on the clinical situation.

1. https://www.cdc.gov>fungal>dieases>candidiasis.
2. https://my.clevelandclinic.org>health.diseases>22.
3. https://www.ncbi.nim.nih.gov>books>NBK560624.

Candida auris (C. auris) is "an emerging multi-drug resistant, yeast-type fungus, found in over 30 countries, was identified as causing the first case of infection in New York state in 2016. [1,2]

It was first identified in 2009 in Japan. [1,2]

Although 'auris' is Latin for ear, it can grow, colonize on skin, in urine, contaminate bed clothing and other surfaces for several weeks and can spread from persons-to-persons.

Symptoms include fever, chills, headaches and low blood pressure.

The mortality rates in persons infected, as opposed to being colonized on the skin is between 30 and 60 %.

People who have invasive disease usually have some underlying disease, or long hospitalizations or Nursing Home patients. [3]

"More than 1 in 3 patients die within a month of being diagnosed with invasive C. auris infection." [3]

Effective treatment is with Echinocandins, fungicidal to many fungi, but fungistatic to Aspergillus. [4]

[1].https://www.gavi.org.
[2].htpps://cdc.gov/fundal/candida/auris/identification.html.
[3].https://www.nks.ok>condition>antifungal-medicines.
[4].htpps://www.cdc.gov/fungal/candida-auris/fastsheets/cdc-message-experts.html.

Coccidioidomycosis (Valley Fever *,**)

This fungal organism grows in soil and dry land and the disease is most common in the aged, 60 and over, and those with weakened immune systems and diabetes. In many cases there are no symptoms, however, common symptoms include fever, night sweats, fatigue, muscle aches and a rash, erythema nodosum may be present

The two forms of the fungi that cause Valley Fever, also called 'Cocci', [1], are Coccidioides immitis and Coccioides posadasii. These are most common in individuals 60 years and older and those with weakened immune systems, diabetes and in Black and Filipino communities.

In many cases these may be no symptoms, but some symptoms are fever, night sweats, muscle aches and a rash, Erythema nodosum.

Diagnosis includes blood tests, skin biopsies, Chest x-ray and C-T of the Chest.

Treatment may include Amphotericin B or fluconazole.

Those who develop Valley Fever develop immunity against re-infection and about 5-10% may develop complications such as COPD or an acute respiratory distress syndrome, and 15-30% may develop Community Acquired Pneumonia. [2]

[1].https://www.cdph.cc.gov>cid>cdc>pages>cocci.
[2].My.clevelandclinic.org/health/diseases/17754-valley-fever.
*Kernpublic.com/valley-fever-Kern.
**https://e.wikipedia.org/wiki/Coccidiodes_posadasii.

"Cryptococcus neoformans is a fungus that lives worldwide and is the most common fungus that causes serious world-wide Lung infections.

It may cause meningitis, with neck pain, fever, headache, nausea and vomiting and light sensitivity.

It does not spread from person -to-person, or from animal-to-person". [1]

"Diagnosis is from cultures from blood, urine and Lumbar puncture, Chest-x-ray and CT scan of the Chest.

In some HIV patients with Cryptococcus meningitis, 50% of blood cultures and 80%. of spinal fluid cultures are positive, or Cryptococcal antigen (Cr Ag) may be detected." [2]

"Treatment consists of three phases: Induction, Consolidation and Maintenance therapy and may include Amphotericin B and Flucytosine in consultation with an Infectious Disease Specialist." [3]

1. https://www.cdc.gov.cryptococcus-neoformans.

2. https://merkmanuals.com>professsional>fungi.
3. https://clinicalinfo.hiv.gov>guideddddddlines>cryptococcus.

"Pneumocystis pneumonia (PCP) is a serious Lung infection caused by the fungus Pneumocystis jirovecii. It is most common in individuals with weakened immune systems, HIV/Aids or on prolonged use corticosteroids. It is an air-borne infection and passes from per-to-person. Symptoms include, cough, fever, chills, fatigue and difficulty breathing.

Diagnosis is by sputa exam or bronchiolar lavage and cultures and a blood test for B-D glucan ("Beta-D glucan is a polysaccaride found in the cell wall of barley, oats, bacteria or yeast or fungi". *) or lung biopsy".[1]

Several types of medications may be used for treatment, such as Bactrim, Septra or co-trimoxazole.

[1] htpps://www.cdc.gov/fungal/diseases/pneumocystis-pneumonia/index.html.
*https://www.the-hospatilist-org>article>criticalcare.

The H_5N_1 species of viruses which caused the recent Pandemic Influenza and early Pandemics, deserve special note.

1. 1918-1919, Spanish Flu, 40-50,000 deaths.
2. 1957- 1958, Asian Flu, 2 million deaths.
3. 1967-1968, Hong Kong Flu, 1 million deaths.

Some other viral illnesses of note are:

H_7N_7 and H_3N_8 cause illness in Horses.

1997- In Hong Kong, 18 patients were hospitalized and 6 died from H_1N_5 infections.

2002- Virginia, Shenandoah Valley, following an out break in poultry of H_7N_2, one person had serological evidence of infection.

2003- In Hong Kong, one child was hospitalized, infected with H_9N and recovered.

2003- In New York City, a patient was admitted with respiratory sign and symptoms. Initial tests showed H_1N_1, recovered and discharged. Confirmatory tests showed H_7N_2.

2004- In Canada, H_7N_3 was identified among poultry workers with eye infections in a poultry outbreak.

As of August 31, 2010 the following chart from the World Health Organization (WHO) shows the following reported laboratory confirmed cases of the H_5N_1 Avian Flu with a cast fatality rate (CFR) of 300/500x100=60%.

Cumulative Number of Confirmed Human Cases of Avian Influenza A/(H5N1) Reported to WHO

31 August 2010

Country	2003 cases	2003 Deaths	2004 Cases	2004 deaths	2005 Cases	2005 deaths	2006 Cases	2006 deaths	2007 cases	2007 deaths	2008 cases	2008 deaths	2009 cases	2009 deaths	2010 cases	2010 deaths	Total Cases	Total deaths
Azerbaijan	0	0	0	0	0	0	8	5	0	0	0	0	0	0	0	0	8	5
Bangladesh	0	0	0	0	0	0	0	0	0	0	1	0	0	0	0	0	1	0
Cambodia	0	0	0	0	4	4	2	2	1	1	1	0	1	0	1	1	10	8
China	1	1	0	0	8	5	13	8	5	3	4	4	7	4	1	1	39	26
Djibouti	0	0	0	0	0	0	1	0	0	0	0	0	0	0	0	0	1	0
Egypt	0	0	0	0	0	0	18	10	25	9	8	4	39	4	22	9	112	36
Indonesia	0	0	0	0	20	13	55	45	42	37	24	20	21	19	6	5	168	139
Iraq	0	0	0	0	0	0	3	2	0	0	0	0	0	0	0	0	3	2

Lao People's Democratic Republic	0	0	0	0	0	0	0	0	2	2	0	0	0	0	0	0	2	2
Myanmar	0	0	0	0	0	0	0	0	1	0	0	0	0	0	0	0	1	0
Nigeria	0	0	0	0	0	0	0	0	1	1	0	0	0	0	0	0	1	1
Pakistan	0	0	0	0	0	0	0	0	3	1	0	0	0	0	0	0	3	1
Thailand	0	0	17	12	5	2	3	3	0	0	0	0	0	0	0	0	25	17
Turkey	0	0	0	0	0	0	12	4	0	0	0	0	0	0	0	0	12	4
Viet Nam	3	3	29	20	61	19	0	0	8	5	6	5	5	5	7	2	119	59
Total	4	4	46	32	98	43	115	79	88	59	44	33	73	32	37	18	505	300

Total number of cases includes number of deaths. WHO reports only laboratory-confirmed cases. All dates refer to onset of illness. Indonesia numbers indicate cumulative total of sporadic cases and deaths which occurred during 2009.

The above Table has since been modified numerous times during the writing of this book.

Malaria (M)

The word Malaria is derived from the Italian word mala aria *"bad air"*, and was once called ague or Marsh Fever.

The British Physician Ronald Ross was awarded the Nobel Prize in 1902 for his work on Malaria.

In 2015, the Chinese Researcher TuYou was awarded the Nobel prize for her work on the anti-malarial drugs Artemisinin and Artesunate. These have anti-pyretic properties, fever reducing, as shown by the drug Artesunate which is water soluble for oral, rectal, intra muscular or intra venous administration. (a,aa)

Malaria is a disease caused by a Parasite that infects a mosquito, usually the female Anopheles, a night biting insect, between dusk and dawn, then at some point bites a person.

The Parasites are Plasmodium falciparum, vivax, ovale, malariae and knowlesi. Plasmodium falciparum, the most common, causes the most deaths. P. vivax is the milder form, seen in South America. P. ovale is uncommon, primarily located in West Africa; resides in the liver for years without causing symptoms. P. malariae is rare, seen only in Africa and knowlesi, also rare, seen in South East Asia.

Birds and non-human primates are also infected by the Plasmodium species. (s,ss)

There are about 1,7000 cases in America yearly with over 215 million cases world-wide and more than 700,000deaths.

Symptoms include a "flu-like" illness, chills and high fevers and sweating. Other signs and symptoms may include headache, nausea and vomiting and diarrhea.

After the bite infection occurs in the liver, the red blood cells (RBC) are invaded. In 48 to 72 hours, the RBC bursts causing the chills, fever and sweating.

Spread can occur through Blood Transfusions, rarely from sharing needles. Spread can occur from mother to infant and in transplants.

There is no known person to person spread.

The incubation period may be from 7 to 30 days. Liver failure causes jaundice with yellowish discoloration of the eyes and skin, pale colored stools and dark colored urine. (j)

Most infections are in three Stages:

Cold Stage---sensation of cold and shivering.

Hot Stage----fever, headache, vomiting, seizures in young children.

Sweating Stage---tiredness, sweating, return to normal temperatures.

with blood tests.

The *gold standard* for diagnosis is the microscopic exam of the cells which shows the parasite.

The first effective treatment for Malaria was from quinine, from the bark of the cinchona tree.

Effective treatment now includes the anti-malaria drugs, the anti-pyretic drug, Artemisinin and Spraying (DEET N, N-diethyl-meta -toluamide) and Nets. (d, Rx).

The mortality rate for Malaria world- wide is between 1-3 million deaths per year. It is the fourth leading cause of death in children under 5 years of age. (de).

Other causes of death in children under 5 years and younger include Prematurity, acute infections, pneumonia and diarrhea and birth trauma and asphyxia. (q)

As of 2015 the Vaccine RTS, S/AS01 (ROI), to be used in 2019, was approved for young children in four doses, against P. falciparum "in regions with moderate to high transmission". *,**

Anti-Malaria meds include quinolones and primaquine.

All treatment for Malaria should be directed by Infectious Disease Specialists.

(m) Malaria-en.wikipedia.org>wiki>malaria.
* https://www.int.>News>item
**cdc.gov/parasites/features/malaria_vaccine_who.html.
(a) www.britannica.com/science/atremisinin

Carabello, H (2014), Emergency Department Management of Mosquito-borne illness, Malaria, Dengue West Nile virus, Emergency Medicine. Practice 16 (5) Archived from the original on 2016-08-01.

(aa) en.wikipedia.org/wiki/artemisinin.

(de) www.medscape.ccom/answers/221134-407901/what-is.

(d) https://www.epa.gov/insect-repellents/deet.

(d) WHO 77, Indoor Residual Spraying for Scaling Up Global Malaria Control and Elimination; WHO Position Statement (PDF) (Report)

WHO 2006 Archived (PDF) from the original0n 2008-10-02.

(q) quizlet.com/13770929/Chapter -10-thehealth-of.

(rx) WHO (2010) Guidelines for the treatment of Malaria (PDF)

(Report) (2nd.ed) World Health Organization.

ISBN 978-92-4-152792-5.

(s) Annals of the New York Academy of Sciences, 1249:211-26

doi:10.11/J.1749-6632.2011. 06431.y PMid223220256.

(ss) Ameri, M (2010), "Laboratory diagnosis of Malaria in non-Human Primates", Veterinary Clinical Pathology 39 (1): 5-

19.doi:10.1111/J.1939-165x.2010.00217x PMID 20456124.

www.malariavaccine.org
https://www.who.int/news-room/fact-sheets/detail/monkeypox

Mad Cow Disease

Also known as Bovine Spongiform Encephalopathy (BSE) is a progressive neurological disorder affecting cattle, due to infection from a transmissible agent called a *prion*.

According to the CDC, "the term prion refers to abnormal, pathogenic agents that are transmissible and are able to induce abnormal folding of specific normal cellular proteins called prion proteins that are found most abundantly in the brain". *

Some other human related prion diseases are Creuzfeldt-Jakob Disease (CJD) and a variant called vCJD (Variant Creutzfeldt-Jakob Disease).

Normal functions of these proteins are not completely understood. The abnormal foldings lead to brain damage, usually rapidly progressive and always fatal.

The CDC identifies them as transmissible spongiform encephalopathies (TSEs)."

Common human forms are Cruetzfeltd-Jakob Disease (CJD) and KURU and animal forms are Bovine Spongiform Encephalopathy (BSE), also known as Mad Cow Disease and Chronic Wasting Disease (CWD) which affect deer, elk and moose.

National Institutes of Health: Detecting Human Prion Disease.

The Public Health Impact of Prion Diseases [PDF-191KB]

Transmissible Spongiform Encephalopathies in Humans. [PDF-183KB]

Belay E. Ann. Rev. Microbiol.,1999;53:283-314.

Bovine Spongiform Encephalopathy (BSE), or Mad Cow Disease Resource.

*www.cdc.gov/prions/bse.

Publications related to the Public Health Impact of Prion Diseases (PDF-191KB) are:

Belaay E., Schonberger L., Ann Rev. Public Health2005; 26:191-212.
Belay E. Ann Rev. Microbiol.1999; 53:283-314.

Another agent which deserves special consideration is the multi drug resistant tuberculosis organism (MDRT) especially in an increasingly immune-compromised population world-wide.

Bioterrorism: Guidelines for Medical and Public Health Management, Henderson, Inglesby, O'Toole, JAMA and Archives Journals, 2002 by the American Medical Association.

A number of other newly emerging infectious diseases have been noted in the United States and world-wide in the 21st Century, such as Covid-19, discussed elsewhere, and Monkey pox, also classified as a world-wide Emergency in July 2022.

MONKEY P0X (MPox) (this information is primarily from the World Health Organization [who, mp]).

M-Pox is now the preferred name.

Monkey Pox is a rare viral zoonotic disease transmitted to humans from animals such as Gambian giant rats and squirrels in Africa, and in America from Prairie dogs.

The first identified case of human Monkey Pox was in 1970 in a 9-year-old boy in Zaire and in 1996-97, there was a major outbreak in the Democratic Republic Congo (Zaire). Most of the early cases appear in men who have had sex with men, but no definite link has been established. *

The incubation period ranges from 5 to 21 days.

Signs and symptoms include a rash, lymphadenopathy, fever, intense headache, myalgia and lack of energy. The rash begin in the face and spreads to the palms of the hands and soles of the feet, much like Small Pox.

In addition to the clinical differential which includes chicken pox, measles, syphilis and small pox, blood and serum tests, although these can be inclusive.

Infection can occur from direct contact with bodily fluids from infected animals or eating inadequately cooked meat from infected animals. Congenital Monkey pox can occur with Placental transmission.

As of May 2022, WHO reports "about 6,000 cases annually and 3,000 cases in Nigeria.

In the USA, as of July 6, 2022, there have been 128 confirmed cases of orthopoxvirus/monkey pox virus". (mp)

"Vaccines against Small pox are effective in preventing Monkey pox and in July 2021, CDC reports that Jynneos[tm] (Imvanex) was licensed in the United States." **

Case fatality in Monkey Pox outbreaks is between one and ten percent with most deaths in the young.

As of July 2022, there are over 1,800 cases in the USA according to local news media and WHO has declared it to be a Global Emergency.

*aol.com/newa/expert-monkeypox-likely-spread-sex-092239103-16173313.html.
**https://www.cdc/gov/poxvirus/monkeypox/clinicans/treatment.htm
(mp) https://www.health.ny.gov>press>releases>2022

Shingles, a viral infection that can appear anywhere on the body and causes a painful rash is noted here because it is caused by the varicella-zoster virus, the same virus which causes chicken-pox, and is a member of the orthopoxviral family, which also includes MPox and Small pox, also caused by the varicella virus.

The vaccine against Shingles is RSV Shingrix.

CHAPTER 5

CHEMICAL AGENTS

"Most of the trouble in the world is caused by
people wanting to be important".
T.S. Elliot

Toxic Industrial Chemical (TICS)

Chemical substances which can make individuals ineffective or unable to perform under normal circumstances. The route of exposure may be via inhalation, ingestion or absorption through the skin.

Toxic Industrial Materials (TIMS)

Substances which if exposed too in a given quantity, will produce toxic effects to individuals via inhalation, ingestion, or absorption through the skin.

The three most common Industrial Chemical Agents of concern to the health care provider are Chlorine, Phosgene, and Anhydrous Ammonia NH_3.

These are pulmonary agents which irritate the mucous membranes of the eyes, oro-pharynx, larynx and respiratory tract. Acute and delayed lung injury may occur with bronchospasms and pulmonary edema.

The pungent odor of ammonia is characteristic.

Chemical evaluation initially will include the pulse oximeter, arterial blood gases and a base line chest X-ray. Early intubation and possible Swann-Ganz insertion should be considered as well aggressive fluid monitoring.

Enteral Nutrition or Total Parenteral Nutrition (TPN) may be required.

Whereas it is assumed that healthcare workers in Occupational Medicine are familiar with Cyanide and Fumigants, in this era of bioterrorism the average healthcare provider should likewise have some familiarity.

Examples of highly hazardous TICs are Ammonia, Chlorine, Hydrogen Chloride and Phosgene which are tissue irritants. Some which are systemic poisonous are Arsine, Cyanide, and Hydrogen Sulfide.

Other agents which are less hazardous include carbon monoxide, methyl bromide, arsenic trichloride, parathion and tetraethyl lead.

In terms of the LD_{50} (mg/kg) the most lethal toxin is Botulinum (0.00001 mg/kg). Others for comparison are Nicotene1mg/.kg, Morphine 900mg/kg and Ethanol 10,000mg/kg.

Is there a need to be concerned about TICs and TIM's?

Over 800,000 US businesses use, produce or store TIC's and TIM's. These include airports, college laboratories, farm and garden supply facilities, glass plants, and toxic waste dumps.

Other major sources are photographic suppliers, medical facilities, railroads and tankers which transport propane and other chemicals through major cities.

Various methods of delivering of toxic agents by terrorist organizations could include food water, aerosols, spray, mail, letters, product tempering, and injections.

The challenges presented to the health care provider from chemical agents are no less daunting than from biological or viral agents. Immediate signs or symptoms may be mild or nonexistent, flu like symptoms or gastroenteritis.

Nerve Agents

An article in the Editorial section of the Washington Post Newspaper dated Thursday July 19, 2012 entitled "Unnerving Agents", noted that Syria has a large stockpile of chemical weapons composed of blister and nerve agents including Sarin and VX. It notes also that Syria has prepared chemical weapons for use with SCUD * and SS-21 missiles.

It is important also to note that Syria never signed the 1993 Chemical Weapon's Convention Agreement.

It is estimated that one drop of Sarin can kill an adult and this was the agent used by the Aum Shinrika (Supreme Truth) Cult in the 1995 Tokyo Subway release, affecting 6,000 individuals, killing 12.

A particularly important public health fact with this incident was that of those 6000 affected, "some 1000 to 1,500 self-referred to local Hospitals' and were classified after evaluation as the worried well," as there were no organic findings at the time of the medical evaluation.

*https://en.wikipedia.org>wiki>Scud.

The Classes of Chemical Agents are: [1]

A. Choking---Chlorine, Phosgene, Ammonia (NH_3)

> Absorption through lungs, fluid builds in the lungs and choking victims. Dispersal Gas.

B. Blister—(Vesicants) Mustard Gas, Lewisite.

> Absorption through lungs, skin, burns skin, eyes, blisters.
> Dispersal liquid, aerosol and vapor.

C. Blood—Cyanide.

> Absorption through lungs, oxygen deprivation.
> Dispersal Gas.

D. Nerve Agents (see below).

> Lungs, G series (G=German), skin VX, (V=Venomous),
> paralyzes muscles, seizures, death in 5 minutes or less.
> Dispersal liquid, aerosol, vapor.

E. Riot Control agents—Tear Gas (Mace) CS or CN

> Gas, Eyes, skin, lungs. Fatal in concentrated doses.
> Dispersal Gas.

F. Incapacitants—LSD, BZ, PCP.

> Ingested, psychotic disorders, disorientation.

G. Defoliants—Agent Orange. Paraquat.

> Destroys crops, can cause nerve damage.

> Aerosol. White Phosphorous is often used as a Tracer
> during War time but can burn/melt skin.

1. http://www.opc.org

This type of real-life experiences helps shape the healthcare response in terms of preparation, response, recovery and mitigation for future events.

Nerve agents are the most toxic and rapidly acting of the known chemical warfare agents. They are similar to insecticide pesticides called organophosphates.

Aging is a biochemical process by which the agent...enzyme complex, become refractory to oxime reactivation of the enzyme. For most Nerve Agents the aging time is longer than the time which acute casualties will be seen.

VX has the longest aging process, 24 hours, while Soman is 5 to 8 hours. *

*Fas.org>usa>doctrine>army>mmcch>Nerve Agents.

Soman is a man-made chemical agent developed in Germany in 1930 as an insecticide, also known as "GD".

Vx, the most potent of all nerve agents, was originally developed in the United Kingdom (UK) in the early 1950s. It is an oily liquid odorless and tasteless, amber in color. Symptoms appear within a few seconds after exposure to the vapor form and within minutes, up to 18 hours, after exposure to the liquid form.

Half-lives for the different nerve agents are:

Tabun (GA)----14 hours
Sarin (GB)------5 hours
Soman (GD)—2-6 minutes
Vx-----48 hours

In terms of lethality, VX>GD>GB>GA.

The half-life ($t_{1/2}$) is the time required for a quantity to reduce to half of its initial value. **

**www.en.wikipedia.org/wiki/Half-life.

Two common acronyms useful in dealing with the signs and symptoms of Nerve Agents are DUMBELS and SLUDGE:

DUMBELS SLUDGE

Diarrhea	Salivation
Urination	Lacrimation
Miosis	Urination
Bronchorrhea	Defecation
Emesis	Gastrointestinal
Lacrimation	Emesis

Salivation

These represent the effects on muscarinic receptors, i.e., smooth muscles and glands and the nicotinic receptors i.e., skeletal muscles and ganglia.

Nerve agents block the enzyme acetylcholinesterase (Ache) normally responsible for breaking down acetyl choline (Ach), a neurotransmitter to glands and smooth muscles. When blocked, Ach remains in syncope causing glands to continue to secrete and muscles to contract.

Unless the process is interrupted in a timely manner death may result from lack of oxygen (hypoxia).

Immediate responses are to evacuate the toxic area, if possible, remove all contaminated clothing and make use of available antidotes.

Current devices for employing the Nerve Agent antidotes are the Mark-1, dual injection Kit and the single shot injection Kit. The Antidote Treatment-Nerve Agent, Auto-Injector (ATNAA) is the single shot injector and administers 2.1 mg atropine and 600 mg pralidoxime chloride through a single needle, a time saving sequence of 25 seconds, and has essentially replaced the Mark-1 kit.

Atropine given first helps maintain airway support and dries secretions and 2-PAM removes the agent from the enzyme Ache, allowing restoration functions of Ach.

Diazepam (Valium) treats the resulting seizures from over activity of the muscles. This is available as the Convulsant Antidote for Nerve Agent (CANA) Auto-injector containing 10 mg of diazepam, approved for non-military use since September 29, 2006.

On June 20, 2003 the Atropen (atropine autoinjector) was approved for use in children and adolescents…it had been approved for adults in 1973.

The recommended doses were:

0.5 mg for children weighing between 15 and 40 pounds.
1 mg for children weighing between 40 and 90 pounds.
2 mg doses for adults and children weighing over 90 pounds.

It is important to remember that children and adults do not respond the same for Nerve Agent (NA) poisoning. "Children may respond with neurologic deficits alone, and not with miosis or glandular secretions". (*peds)

Respiratory failure is the primary cause of death in NA- exposed victims. The relationship between concentration and time underscores the need to rapidly evacuate to a vapor-free environment. A child's smaller mass alone reduces the dose of NA required to cause observable and lethal effects. With a higher respiratory rate and minute and volumes than an adult, a child will inhale a greater dose of NA at a constant concentration of toxic vapor. Infants and children are more seizure prone than adults.

The highest incidence of seizures is observed in the first year of life and the greatest incidence of status epilepticus in the first 2 years. It should be intuitive that there are compelling medical and behavioral reasons to establish pediatric-specific zones at the scene of the chemical attack/event.

The pillars of therapy for any NA event/casualty include: intensive respiratory care, antidotal therapy, treatment of complications and long-term monitoring".

(*peds) http://pediatrics.aapublications.org/cgi/content/full/112/3/648

Appropriately trained personnel with appropriate PPE should be safe.

Depending upon the scenario, the average healthcare provider would not encounter a contaminated individual, this having been dealt with at the various early Triage sites.

Contact information for Toxic Agents Regional Poison Control Center (1-800-222-1222).

Convention Agreement.

RICIN (May be considered as a biological agent, was previously discussed in Chapter 4, here-in as an updated incident in October, 2003).

A classic case is that of a 49-year-old male, who suddenly developed leg pain from an apparently accidental injury to his leg from an umbrella while awaiting a bus. Within 15-28 hours he developed nausea, vomiting and fever and he was admitted to the hospital. Within 36 hours increasing fever, tachycardia and lymph node swelling developed and at 48 hours, hypertension and shock developed, despite medical attempts at resuscitation.

By 72 hours anemia had developed, as had hematemesis and cardiac failure, and by hour 84 he was pronounced dead; presumed cause of death, Septic Shock.

At autopsy a "pellet" removed from his leg turned out to be Ricin and follow up investigations would reveal that Gregor Markov, a Belgian Journalist was assassinated by injection from an umbrella. *

Ricin is a compound from the castor bean plant (Ricinnus communis) a commercial source of castor oil. Patho-physiologically, it acts as a cellular toxin which blocks protein synthesis via modification of ribosomal 28s subunit.

Routes of exposure are inhalation, ingestion and parenterally.

The LD_{50} for ricin is 0.05mg/kg, about the size of the head of a pin. There are no known antidotes for ricin toxicity, and only supportive measures for management are available.

On October 22, 2003 ricin was found in a US Postal facility in the District of Columbia, later found to have originated from Greenville, South Carolina and the author, at that time the Medical Director for the Emergency Medical Health Service Administration (EMHSA) of the District of Columbia Department of Health called a midnight teleconference with various Public Health Professionals from the DC, Maryland and Virginia to discuss the event.

There were no health care events associated with the agent, nor with any other incidents in DC with which the author would be involved.

*https://en.wikipedia.org>wiki: Gregor Markov.

The three most common Industrial Chemical Agents of concern to the health care provider are Chlorine, Phosgene, and Anhydrous Ammonia NH_3, as previously noted.

These are pulmonary agents which irritate the mucous membranes of the eyes, oro-pharynx, larynx and respiratory tract. Acute and delayed lung injury may occur with bronchospasms and pulmonary edema.

The pungent odor of ammonia is characteristic.

Chemical evaluation initially will include the pulse oximeter, arterial blood gases and a base line chest X-ray. Early intubation and possible Swann-Ganz insertion should be considered as well aggressive fluid monitoring.

Enteral Nutrition or Total Parenteral Nutrition (TPN) may be required.

Whereas it is assumed that healthcare workers in Occupational Medicine are familiar with Cyanide and Fumigants, in this era of bioterrorism the average healthcare provider should likewise have some familiarity.

Cyanide is rapidly absorbed by inhalation through mucous membranes and by ingestion. Small doses may cause no symptoms, however large or toxic doses may lead to convulsions, coma and death within one to two minutes.

Gradual exposure may be from Hydrogen cyanide gas or the salt form such as Potassium cyanide, sodium or Calcium Cyanide.

Cyanide prevents cells from getting and utilizing oxygen.

Some reported clues or aids in diagnosing cyanide poisoning are the gradual or rapid collapse of an otherwise healthy individual, Hypotension, tachycardia, bradycardia, pink or brightened skin or blood and an odor of "bitter almonds".

Further, these reports also note that some 25% of individuals involved with known cases of cyanide toxicity fail to detect any odor.

Methemoglobinemia is generally present; however, a high level of suspicion is necessary, depending upon the presenting circumstances.

Antidotes are available in the form of Sodium Nitrite and Thiosulfate for intravenous administration and Amyl Nitrate inhalers. If given within minutes of a known exposure, with adequate fluid resuscitation, survival results can be expected.

Many hospitals may have Cyanide antidote kits which may or may not be readily available.

After the event has occurred the kits may be of little use.

Common fumigants used professionally to kill pests are Vikane (Sulfuryl Flouride) Mehtyl Bromide and Phosphine.

Vikane (Sulfuryl Flouride)

Primarily used in structural fumigations. It is a colorless, odorless, non-flammable gas. 3.5 times heavier than air, and usually it is provided with a tent covering the structure.

A normal air level is <5 parts per meter (ppm).

Low concentrations may cause nausea, vomiting, diarrhea, abdominal pain, hypotension, pulmonary edema and cardiac arrhythmia. High concentrations may cause seizures, rapid onset of collapse and respiratory arrest.

These are signs and symptoms very similar to nerve gas toxicity.

There is no specific treatment for Vikane toxicity.

Hypotension, arrhythmias, and electrolyte abnormalities must be aggressively managed.

Methyl-Bromide (Br-CH$_3$)

Odorless and colorless although very high concentrations may produce a chloroform like odor.

Used for fumigating structures and soil under tarps or tents.

Aeration for at least 72 hours is recommended before occupancy without appropriate personal protective equipment.

Signs and symptoms include agitation, headache, delirium seizures, and coma. Nausea and vomiting are common gastro enteric symptoms and irritation of the skin and mucous membranes and pulmonary edema may occur.

There is no specific treatment therefore early and aggressive seizure control, Lidocaine for ventricular arrythmias, fluids and control of hypotension must be instituted.

Phosphine (PH$_3$)

This is a colorless gas but does have a fish or garlic odor with a relatively low odor threshold of 0.15 ppm.

Commercially it is supplied as Phosphine tablets or granules for commodity fumigation. These are commonly Aluminum Phosphide, Zinc Phosphide and Magnesium Phosphide. The granules are usually fumigated for 3 days and when the tablets combine with water in the air, Phosphine is the end product.

The chemical effects appear to be similar to Cyanide.

Early findings are cardiovascular, tachycardia, bradycardia, hypotension, and ventricular arrhythmias; central nervous system findings are confusion, lethargy, convulsion, and coma.

Delayed toxicity may be manifest as pulmonary edema.

Grain freighters may use Phosphine as a fumigant.

There is no antidote or specific treatment, again requiring aggressive supportive management.

There have been several fatalities reported from Phosphine gas associated with the illegal production of Methamphetamine.

Herbicides used by the Military included Agents White and Agent Blue, used in large scale as an anti-crop agent.

Other colors, green and purple were also used but were soon dropped.

En.wikipedia.org>wiki>Agent_White.

En.wikipedia.org>wiki>Rainbow_Herbicide.

This type of real-life experiences helps shape the healthcare response in terms of preparation, response, recovery and mitigation for future events.

Nerve agents are the most toxic and rapidly acting of the known chemical warfare agents. They are similar to insecticide pesticides called organophosphates.

Soman is a man-made chemical agent developed in Germany in 1930 as an insecticide, also known as "GD".

Vx, the most potent of all nerve agents, was originally developed in the United Kingdom (UK) in the early 1950s. It is an oily liquid odorless and tasteless, amber in color. Symptoms appear within a few seconds after exposure to the vapor form and within minutes, up to 18 hours, after exposure to the liquid form.

"Vx is the most toxic nerve agent available in the West. It is an inhibitor of acetylcholinesterase (ACHE), which acts by increasing the acetylcholine (ACH) at the nerve synapses. Toxicity sets in when more than 50% of the ACHE enzyme is inhibited." *

Depending upon the scenario, the average healthcare provider would not encounter a contaminated individual, this having been dealt with at the various early Triage sites.

Contact information for Toxic Agents Regional Poison Control Center (1-800-222-1222).

Centers for Disease Control and Prevention (CDC)

1-800-232-4636 (English and Spanish).

www.bt.cdc.gov/
cdcinfo@cdc.gov
*htpps://www.ncbi.nim.ih.gob>books>NBK535428

Agency for Toxic Substances and Disease Registry (ATSDR) 1-888-422-8737

atsdric@cdc.gov

What Is a Chemical Weapon?

At various meetings between April 1972 and March 1980, the Chemical Weapons Convention (CWC) and the Biological and Toxin Weapons Convention (BTWC) have formulated a definition for a chemical weapon.

OPCW.
http://www.opc.org

The definition includes three components:

1. All toxic chemicals and their precursors, which can cause death, temporary or permanent harm to humans or animals. Some of these have a dual use, as determined by "The general-purpose criterion". Thus, an agent such as Chlorine is a key component in certain commercial products. A basic component of the criterion is the principle of consistency i.e., the product must be of a type and quantity appropriate for that purpose.
2. The Chemical Weapons includes "any munitions or devices specifically designed to inflict harm or cause death through release

of the toxic chemicals". These could include missiles, bombs, artillery shells or mortars. (Principle of Specificity).

3. Any equipment designed specifically used in direct connection with the munitions noted in #2. The Principle of Specificity applies here also".

Riot control agents (RCAs) are chemical agents but not included in the CWC schedule because the disabling effects usually disappear in a relatively short time.

Toxic chemicals produced by living organisms are also addressed in the Biological and Toxic Weapons Convention (BTWC), however a number of these are dual-use chemicals which are used for legitimate purposes.

One such toxin Ricin (ri), is part of the waste mash produced when castor oil is made, and has been used in some forms of cancer therapy.

Ricin also was identified as the agent used to kill Georgi Markov, a Bulgarian Journalist in 1978 in London, after he was attacked by an individual with an umbrella injected a pellet of Ricin. Within several days he as dead of multiple organ failure and at autopsy, the pellet was discovered.

Ricin was previously discussed however; additional information has surfaced since the earlier discussion.

A 57-year-old male was hospitalized for 3 months in Las Vegas, Nevada from Ricin poisoning, and in March 2014 a 19-year-old male as arrested by the Federal Bureau of Investigation (FBI) and charged with possessing Ricin.

In October 2003, an envelope containing Ricin was found in an airport postal building signed "The Fallen Angel", for whom a $100,000 reward was offered. It is unclear if the individual was ever found.

These accounts of Ricin and for the ATNAA Injector, can be found in a document titled Terrorism for The Clinician: Diagnosis & Treatment of Exposures to Chemical, Radiation & Biotoxins, April & May 2014, pages

2-6, 14-15, 19,20,21 and 40-50, National Capital Poison Center, 3201 New Mexico Ave., NW, Suite 310, Washington, DC, 20016, 1-800-222-1222.

Briefly presented in the document also is a short discussion of the radioactive isotope Polonium-210, which occurs in low levels naturally.

Commercially it is used to prevent static electricity build up.

It was recovered from the exhumed corpse of Yassar Araphat and was thought to be the agent to poison Alexander Litvenenko in November 2006.

The Guradian.com/world/2013/nov/06/polonium-210-poison-alexander-litvinenko.

Data indicates that a 500-microgram dose of Ricin would be about the size of the head of a pin and powerful enough to kill an adult.

It can be found as a powder, pellet or a mist and can be dissolved in water, is generally a stable substance, but can be inhaled, ingested or injected.

Ricin poisoning is not contagious.

Symptoms of Ricin poisoning depend on the route of exposure with difficulty breathing, cough, tightness in the chest occurring within 6 hours or less. Other findings include pulmonary edema, fever, nausea, vomiting bloody diarrhea and low blood pressure. Chest x-ray may show bilateral infiltrates within the first 2-3 days. Leukocytosis is seen and ELISA and PCR tests will be positive.

Along with clinical findings, diagnosis is helped by a rapid urine test, but if positive, must be confirmed be a second test performed by a Laboratory in the Laboratory Response Network (LRN), a CDC Lab.

Components of the castor bean or an assay showing ricinine should be positive for Ricin.

There is no antidote for Ricin poisoning and therapy is primarily supportive.

(ri) www.bt.cdc.gov

Emergency.cdc.gov/ agents>ricin>facts

www.webmd.com First Aid&emergencies>references

Thallium [Th]

Thallium is a chemical agent not found free in nature, but which has been used for poisoning individuals. Historically it has been referred to as "the poisoner's poison" and "inheritance powder" along with arsenic.

It is odorless, colorless and tasteless and has been found in some vegetables, e.g., radish, turnips and spinach.

It can be inhaled as well as absorbed through the skin.

Symptoms of Thallium poisoning include abdominal pain, diarrhea, fever, anorexia, all non-specific. [th1]

Early diagnosis often does not occur and it is not until hair loss, days later that arouse suspicion.

Blood tests with a quantitative atomic absorption will confirm the diagnosis.

Thallium is a product of coal combustion along with slag and ash. Previously it has been used as rat and ant poisoning.

Commercially it is used in manufacturing electric devices and as a nuclear cardiac stress scan.

There is an antidote, Prussian Blue (Radiogardase {TM}), which binds the thallium as does activated charcoal.[th]

[th] en.wikipedia.org>news>thallium_poisoning
[th1] calpoison.org>newsthallium-poisoning
[th2] https://pubmed.ncbi.nim.nih.gov>..

Novichok *

Another Nerve Agent which has been in the news in recent years is Novichok, said to be much more toxic than Sarin on VX, and causing death in 30 seconds to 2 minutes if treatment is not started.

It is the agent alleged to have been used in the poisoning of the former Russian spy Sergei Skriypal and his daughter Yulia.** Likewise it is thought to have been the agent used in the poisoning of the half- brother of Kim Jong Un of North Korea.

It is a binary agent developed in Russia and the Soviet Union in the 1970s and 1980s. It is one of the four binary nerve Agents developed in the past; Sarin (GB2), Soman (GD2) and VX (VX2) are the other three.

"A binary agent is a chemical weapon which contain the toxic agent in its active state as a chemical precursor, significantly less toxic than the agent.

A unary agent contains a single element or one component". *

*Wikidiff.com/una+ry/binary
**https://en.wikipedia.org>wiki>Poisoning_of_Sergei_

Lead

Lead Poisoning is very common, the most significant environmental health problem for children. Lead comes from paint and gasoline- still a problem along highways, solder, and industrial sources such as smelter. Other potential sources of lead in the environment come from lead glazed pottery, brass fittings in well pumps, lead water pipes, home remedies or cosmetics, firing ranges, automotive repair, casting ammunition, fishing weights or sinkers, burning lead painted wood or lead batteries.

The major impact of Lead on the body includes maternal lead levels which may affect pregnancy (preterm labor, lead in the mothers' body, even from her childhood, may cross the placenta and enter the baby).

The historical perspective of lead began in the 1920s introduction of tetraethyl lead as octane booster in gasoline. In the 1940s recognition by Byers and Lord that lead poisoning created long-term sequela in survivors as recorded.

In the 1960s, Chelation was introduced by Julian Chisolm as a means of preventing seizures, coma and death from heavy metals and some Toxins.

Chelation Therapy removes heavy metals, e.g., Lead, Mercury, Arsenic and Toxins. It involves injecting into the blood stream a chemical solution using EDTA (ethylene diamine tetra-acetic acid) which binds with the minerals. There are other agents used as well.

(draxe.com/chelation-therapy, www.verywellhealth-com/what-is-chelation-90006 www.ihealthtube.com /video/how-chelation-mineral-work-body).

In the 1970s and beyond, a decrease in average blood Lead level in children in the United States was reported. In the 1980s and beyond, recognition that Lead levels, previously thought to be acceptable, are in fact, injurious to children's neurocognitive development. In the 1980s recognition of need to find ways of making existing housing stocks lead-free or lead-safe.

In 1980s and 90s activities were under the auspices of or with funding by HUD to decrease lead-based paint in housing.

The use of lead in ancient times for water pipes and utensils in the late 19th century began to be recognized as the cause of medical problems in some parts of the world. In early 20th century the banning of residential use of lead-based paint in some parts of the world began. Throughout the 20th century the obfuscation on the part of the Lead industry about the hazards of lead began.

The impact of lead on the body includes blood lead levels in children being greater than 10-ug/dL with elevated threshold and decreased linear growth. Greater than 10-ug/dL may include learning disabilities and behavior problems.

Children with blood levels that are 20-ug/dL have decreased nerve conduction velocity, 40 ug/dL have decreased hemoglobin synthesis, 80 ug/dL have encephalopathy, seizures or coma, > 100 ug/dL can cause death.

Children are at greatest risks for lead poisoning. One and two-year-old children are at greater risk. Increased mobility during the second year of life, resulting in more access to lead hazards with normal hand to mouth activities, this age group will put anything in their mouths.

Lead is an element which does not degrade in the environment.

The current acceptable blood lead level is 10 ug/dL. The success in lowering lead levels came from decreasing and removing lead from these products, gasoline, paint, cans, water (Lead pipes) and ceramics.

1. www.leadinspector.com
2. www.healthcareknow/com
3. www.mayoclinic.org.diseases-condition/lead-poisoning/symptoms-causes/sye-203544717
4. kidshealth.org/en/parents/lead/poisoning.html

Mercury (Hg)

In October 2003, a student at a local High School here in Washington DC, took a bottle of Mercury from his Chemistry Laboratory at the end of class, and began "showing it around to his friends". He visited a nearby Junior High School where some of the Mercury somehow contaminated a class room, also a friend, and his cat.

At the time I was the Medical Director for The Emergency Health and Medical Services Administration (EHMSA), in the Department of Health here in Washington DC.

We initiated the Unified Command System and working with the Fire Department, the Metropolitan Police Department and the Department of Mental Health, we visited each of the schools which were involved, after having identified the student who as responsible, as well as each of the apartments he had visited, a process which lasted well after midnight.

All of the individuals who were identified as having any contact with the Mercury were relocated to a local Hotel.

One of the most challenging events during the relocation was catching and removing the cat. Dr. Gabriella Gonzales, then Chief of the Emergency Medical Services (EMS) worked closely with us in responding to the Spanish speaking residents.

There were no medical issues ever documented because of the Mercury spill.

Our primary goal then was re-assuring those residents who were exposed, that there was no reason for concern.

As a result of the incident, thermometers which contained Mercury were removed from the schools, and the local community was advised not to use Mercury filled thermometers.

A much more in-depth review of Mercury Poisoning can be found in the various references listed below, and from which much of this information was obtained.

Mercury Poisoning may result from excessive exposure with symptoms due to duration, ingestion or inhalation, depending on the type.

There are three forms of Mercury, Elemental, in liquid form as in glass thermometers, Inorganic, batteries, some disinfectants and Organic, in fish. [6]

They may include numbness of the hands and feet, muscle weakness, anxiety, memory losses, skin rashes and difficulty seeing or hearing.

Children may develop acrodynia (Pink Disease) in which the skin becomes pink and peels. [1]

Most human exposure is from eating fish, although amalgam based dental fillings may still be in circulation, and may be associated with certain occupations such as mining for gold. [2,3]

Prevention includes avoiding mercury containing foods.

The various forms of mercury are vapor, salts, metal and the organic compound. Mining for gold and burning coal may be associated with inhaling mercury.

Blood tests, tests for urine and hair are available for diagnosis. [3]

Acute poisoning may respond to Chelation Therapy. [4,5]

(Hg) https://en.wikipedia.org/wiki/Mercury_poisoning
[1] Horowitz Y, et al., "Acrodynia: a case report of two siblings", (https://www.ncbi.nim.nih/gov/pmc/aarticles/PMC1762992)[2,3]
Bernhoft, RA (2012) "Mercury toxicity and treatment: a review of the literature". (https//www.ncbi.nim.nih/gov/pmc/articles/PMC3253456).
[4,5] "Mercury and Health".
https://www.who.int/mediacentre/factsheets/fs361/en/
[1] Kosnett, MJ (December 20213) "The role of chelation in the treatment of arsenic and mercury poisoning".

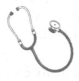

CHAPTER 6 A

BIO-CONTAINMENT LABORATORIES

There are four levels of Biocontainment laboratories.

Biosafety Level 1 (BSL-1).

The average university research lab, i.e., for undergraduate microbiology has few restrictions on who may enter, and is directly connected with the rest of the building; requires wearing of a lab coat and normal lab hygiene practices.

Lab work done on open air bench tops without specialized equipment for microorganisms. Routine safety features exist, e.g., hand washing, no food or drink in the work area, decontamination of work bench tops before and after use. Personnel are trained to prevent contamination of themselves or experiments which may be ongoing.

Biosafety Level 2 (BSL-2)

Similar in design and operation as a BSL 1 facility, however safety features are in place to allow for the study of micro-organisms that are potentially hazardous. Access is restricted and individuals known to have deficient immune systems are not allowed. Specific personnel are trained to handle specific disease-causing organisms and personal protective equipment, e.g., specialized clothes, face masks, sterile gloves are required. Personnel require frequent testing and/or Vaccination. Procedures such as blending and centrifugation are employed creating the opportunity for air borne microorganisms.

There are no specific ventilation system requirements and air enters and exits via the buildings systems.

Biosafety Level 3 (BSL- 3)

This Laboratory works with the microorganisms that can easily become airborne with a high infectivity risk. All work with the microorganisms must be done within biological safety cabinets and by trained personnel in appropriate personal protective equipment. There are increased restrictions for access to the Laboratory.

Newer facilities must have double doors, sealed around the edges and the outer door must be fully closed before the inner door to the lab is opened. Ventilation is independent from the remainder of the facility and the exhaust air is filtered to remove microorganisms. The floor and walls are designed to be impermeable to fluids.

Laboratory personnel and equipment are regularly monitored and deemed safe to function on an annual basis.

Biosafety Level 4 (BSL- 4)

These facilities work with microorganisms which pose a major health threat. They deal with such agents as Small pox, Ebola, Marburg and Lassa viruses and the Bacillus anthracis which causes Anthrax.

Any genetically engineered agents are studied here.

An example are the agents described by Ken Alibek in his book "Biohazard", where in the virus which causes Small pox, variola major, was combined with the Ebola virus to produce *"Black pox"*, most assuredly a fiendish plot!

These agents may be airborne and easily transmitted by air and from person to person being highly infectious.

Anthrax is not transmitted from person to person and it is not contagious. The anthrax organisms may be crystallized and delivered as an airborne agent. This capability recently discovered from information discovered in Iraq, was the impetus this country developing the City Readiness Plan.

This plan will be discussed in another chapter (see Chapter 11).

As of 2002, BSL- 4 facilities in North America are located at the United States Army Research Institute of Infectious Disease (USAMRIID) in Fort Detrick, Maryland, the CDC in Atlanta, Georgia, San Antonio, and Winnipeg, Manitoba, Canada.

Another facility is planned for the National Institute of Allergy and Infectious Diseases Rock Mountain Lab in Hamilton, Montana.

Personnel are highly trained and expert in microbiological techniques and have been vaccinated against the agents with which they will be working.

All work is done in Level A facilities with personnel protective equipment.

The laboratory is completely isolated from the remainder of the rooms in the building and I reverse osmosis filtration system is in place. All the work in the laboratory is documented.

The new facility planned for Hamilton, Montana will be fenced in and guarded as well as being equipped with cameras and multi levels of secured access; and the exteriors will be completely illuminated at night.

www.esponiageinfo.com/Ba-B1/Biocontainment-laboratories.html

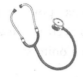

CHAPTER 6 B

THE BIO-WATCH PROGRAM

This is a system designed to detect the release of pathogens into the air there by providing warning to the public health community, local and federal government of a potential biological bioterrorism event.

It is based in great part by the Biological Aerosol Sentry and Information System (BASIS), developed by scientists at Lawrence Livermore and Los Alamos National Laboratories. The program is funded by the Department of Homeland Security (DHS) and has three primary elements, sampling, analysis, and response, each coordinated by different agencies. The Environmental Protection Agency (EPA) maintain the sampling component, sensors which collect airborne particles; the Centers for Disease Protection (CDC) coordinates the analyses via a Nationwide laboratory Response Network of over 118 labs and local jurisdictions which are responsible for the Public Health Response.

The Federal Bureau of Investigation is the lead agency for law enforcement if a bioterrorist event is detected.

The sensor network is ongoing in over 30 cities in the United States. The filters are collected at regular 24 hours intervals and analyzed for potential pathogens using Polymerase Chain Reaction (PCR) techniques.

With early notifications of a bioterrorism event, it is assumed by public health authorities, this will provide some advantage in prevention and treatment.

Current news reports indicate that some of the pathogens which can be detected are anthrax, plague, small pox, and tularemia. For safety reasons, the Department of Homeland Security does not list all the pathogens or the locations of the Bio-watch monitors.

The system was first deployed for both indoor and outdoor monitoring at the Salt Lake City, Utah Olympics in 2002.

The exact costs are not provided however it was estimated by the Associated Press in 2003 that the installation costs were $1 million per city with a yearly operations budget of $ 1 million per city.

A list of some 96 references can be obtained at:

http://www.far.org/sgp/os/terror/RL32152.html

According to an article in the Washington Post Newspaper, page A15, July 16, 2008 the Bio-watch Program which is now 5 years old and operational in over 30 large US cities, including Washington, D.C., still lack basic technical data to help medical officials how to respond to an alert triggered by the sensors.

The article further states that written testimony submitted for a House hearing on July 16, 2008, state and local public health laboratory directors were highly critical of the program, saying it was under-funded, improperly managed and of unclear benefit, despite $ 400 million in federal spending.

In addition to the Bio-watch system, there is under development an Autonomous Detection System (ADS), to detect biological and chemical agents in the environment. This system is designed to provide reliable alerts for the presence of a biological or chemical hazard.

The existing Autonomous Detection System tests for the Bacillus anthracis organism which causes Anthrax, and is in place in many US Postal distribution centers.

If an aerosolized Bacillus anthracis spore in an air sample is identified, immediate onsite decontamination and evacuation at the facility can occur.

A report by the CDC in its Morbidity and Mortality Weekly Report (MMWR), June 4, 2004/53(RR07);1-12, discusses this system in great detail. *

In March, 2005, the Author was one of the physicians from the District of Columbia Department of Public Health ESF #8 response group which was alerted when a positive anthrax alarm was received from the Curseen/Morrris Postal Facility in Washington, DC. This was the previous Brentwood facility where the original anthrax organisms were identified in October 2001, which infected 5 postal workers, two of whom Joseph Curseen Jr., 47, and Thomas Morris Jr. 55, died, previously discussed.

These were the two workers for whom the facility was renamed.

Another worker Leroy Richmond contracted anthrax at the facility in 2001 but he survived. (See Newspaper article).

He was one of the individuals interviewed by the FBI following the apparent suicide of the Microbiologist Bruce E. Ivins who worked at the Lab in Fort Detrick, Md., and has been held responsible for the anthrax attack.

Numerous articles in the Washington Post and New York Times discussed many of the details of the incident. The Justice Department had earlier dismissed their case against Dr. Stephen Hatfield, "a person of interest" and had settled a legal claim with him of some $5,800,000 million dollars

*http://www.cdc.gov/mmwr/preview/mmwrhtml/rr530al.htm

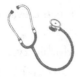

CHAPTER 7

RADIOLOGICAL AND NUCLEAR AGENTS

"The means by which we live have outdistanced the ends for which we live. Our scientific power has outrun our spiritual power. We have guided missiles and misguided men."

Martin Luther King Jr.

Macrina Wiedrekehr, O.S.B. A Tree Full of Angels.

Radioactivity is generally not well understood by many healthcare providers, whether from a nuclear detonation or a Dirty Bomb.

The detonation of a nuclear device of 1-kiloton (1000 kg of tri-nitro-toluene [TNT]*), 2-methyl-1, 3, 5-Trinitro benzene] would be associated with massive physical injuries, many irradiated casualties and down-wind fallout of radioactive contamination.

*(en.Wikipedia.org/wiki/Trinitrotoluene).

The force of the explosion would be comparable to the device used to bomb Japan in World War II.

"On August 6 and 9th, 1945 two nuclear weapons were detonated over the Japanese cities of Hiroshima and Nagasaki, killing over 200,000 thousand people.

"The discovery by Nuclear Physicists in a Laboratory in Berlin, Germany in 1938, made the first atomic bomb possible, after Otto Hahn, Lise Meitner and Fritz Strassman, discovered nuclear fission". [1]

[1] htpps://www.sciencehistory.org>historical-profile>ott.

Dr. J. Robert Oppenheimer is considered as "The Father of the Atomic Bomb". [2,3]

[2] https//wwww.history.com>topics>world-war- II>atomic.
[3] https/en.wikipedia.org>J_Robert_Oppenheimer.

Also, just as important, Lise Meitner, is considered "The Mother of the Atomic Bomb". [4]

[4] https://www.dw.com>lise-meitner-mother-of-the-atomic-bomb.

During the final stages of World War II, the United States and its allies had called for an unconditional surrender of the Imperial Japanese Armed Forces, responsible for the bombing of Pearl Harbor, December 7, 1941 in the Potsdam Declaration on July 26, 1941.

The alternative was prompt and utter destruction!

Japan ignored the ultimatum and the war continued. By August of 1945, the Allies Manhattan Project had produced two types of Atomic Bombs.

On August 6, 1945, a modified B-29 Bomber dropped a Uranium -235-gun-type (Little Boy) on Hiroshima. On August 9, 1945 a Plutonium -238 implosion-type (Fat Man) nuclear bomb was dropped over Nagasaki. [atp]

Estimates of 46% of deaths from Leukemia in Japan during the period 1950 to 2000 were attributed to the bombings and 11% of Solid tumors.

A hypothetical scenario put forth involves "the six cities most likely to be hit by a Nuclear Bomb, Washington DC, New York City, Chicago Illinois, Houston Texas, Los Angeles California and San Francisco California".[5]

Alex Wellerstein, a nuclear weapons historian, has developed an interactive tool, the Nuke Map, which given certain areas, one can simulate some of the consequences of a city hit by a 15-kiloton explosion like the one that detonated over Hiroshima during World War II. [6]

Simulation projected "New York city would sustain 225 thousand deaths and 610 thousand injuries, Washington DC, 120 thousand deaths, 169 injuries, and Los Angeles California100 thousand deaths and 151 thousand injuries."

"As of 2022, the Federation of American Scientists estimates Russia possesses 5,977 nuclear weapons, while the United States has 5,428; Russia and the U.S. each have about 1,600 active deployed strategic nuclear war heads." [7]

A key to help with understanding the Nuke Map tool is the following color code:

"Yellow: A fireball (590-foot radius), less than one-millionth of one second after the explosion.

Green: Radiation (0.74 miles radius), within 15 minutes radioactive particles and nuclear fall-out would reach the ground.

Blue-Grey: Air blast (1.04 miles radius).

Orange: Thermal radiation (1.18) mile radius. All healthcare facilities in the area would be completely overwhelmed." [8]

"Dirty Bomb", [db] or Radiological Diversion Device (RADD), is a conventional explosive device using TNT and some radioactive element e.g., Iodine 131 or Cesium 137.

The primary injuries would result from the explosion over the immediate area, but the greater effect would be from the radioactive material the device carries to those exposed, victims and rescue personnel and possibly victims at distant sites, down-wind from the primary explosion.

The psychological consequences of such an explosion may well lead to significant social disruption.

Another scenario requiring less sophistication would be the release of radiation particles in liquid or gas form which could contaminate public space or drinking water, as might occur from a spray or aircraft. It is likely that the amount of radioactivity small with little physical harm from acute radiation; however, the psychological impact again would be quite large.

Basically, isotopes are any of the forms of a chemical element that differ in the number of neutrons in an atomic particle, nearly equal in mass to the proton.

A proton is a positively charged atomic particle present in all atomic nuclei, the electron being the negatively charged particle.

Isotopes may be stable or unstable. Unstable isotopes undergo decay and emit electromagnetic radioactivity such as x-rays, gamma rays, alpha and beta rays or neutrons, or combinations of each different type of unstable isotope. As the emitted radioactivity proceeds along pathways, energy is transferred into the medium, viz, air, liquids, until there is complete dissipation of the energy.

When radiation proceeds through tissue, resulting in ionization or the production of free radicals of oxygen or water in the cell, these free radicals may result in immediate and long-term injury to the cell.

The units of measurements of radiation are shown below.

The severity and rate of acute radiation injury are directly related to the dose and time (duration) of exposure.

Exposure greater than 1 gray unit (Gy) may occur from an actual nuclear explosion, unlike that which would occur from a conventional (TNT) or dirty bomb. Long term effects or carcinogenic effects would occur years later after a prolonged latent period, e.g., Leukemia or Solid Tumors after 20-30 years.

Medical management of a Dirty Bomb generally entails decontamination at the explosion site with thorough cleaning of the individuals, removal of clothing and appropriate eye care.

Any trauma from the explosion is cared for as would any major trauma.

The Radiation exposure is generally not considered a major result however, that decision must rest with the local Healthcare Departments.

A Nuclear detonation of a 1-kiloton device would have a Lethal Dose radius [LD_{50}] of approximately 50% of those exposed of about 300 miles in all directions from the blast. Thermal injury may well have a LD_{50} of 600 miles and multiple blast injuries from debris, glass and fires would occur.

An early account of exposure to a Dirty Bomb come from Goinia, Brazil, September 1987 –March 1988. *

A capsule was removed from an abandoned Radiotherapy Clinic for Teletherapy, the source containing powdered Cesium -137. The plan was to sell the capsule as scrap metal. Later that day, both men developed nausea, vomiting, diarrhea and a swollen hand, thought to be signs of acute radiation illness.

A few days later, one of the men punctures the Capsule and the powder leaked out. Realizing the powder glowed blue, he took it to his family and friends to see.

After 2 weeks of contact with the substance increasing numbers of people were showing adverse health effects. By this time, 240 people were contaminated and 151 showed external and internal effects, with 20 individuals becoming seriously ill and 5 died.

According to the Nuclear Regulatory Commission, there are nine reactor isotopes produces isotopes which may be suitable for radiological terror.

Americum-241, Californium-252, Cesium-137, Cobalt-60, Irrridum-192, Plutonium-238, Polonium-210, Radium-226, and Strontium-90.

Wikipedia Foundation.

db https://en.wikipedia.org.wiki>Dirty bomb.
* http://en.wikipedia.org/wiki/dirty bomb.

It appears that the idea behind a dirty bomb is to blast radioactive material into the explosion, possible exposing people and buildings. The main purpose is to frighten people and make buildings and land unsafe for some period of time.

Radiation cannot be seen, smelled, tasted or felt by humans.

One of the radiation sources in a Dirty Bomb may be Iodine -131. If this source is suspected, Potassium Iodide (KI) can be used to protect the persons Thyroid Gland from injury.

atbhttps://en.wikipedia.org/wiki/Atomic bombing of Hiroshimia and Nagasaki
[2]www.national terroralert.com/dirty-bomb/Dirty Bomb Emergency Kit.
[1,3] https://www.nukepills.com/dirty-bomb-emergrncy-kit/Prussian Blue has been proven effective for ingestion of Cesium-147.
[4] https://www.nrc.gov/reading-rm/dc-collection/fact sheets/fs dirtybomb html
[5] Newsletter3@trendingg4now.com
[6] Nuclearsecrecy.com/NukeMap.
[7] https://alexwellerstein.com>projects>nukemao
[8] https:worldwidepopulationsreview.com>country-rankins.

CHAPTER 8

EXPLOSIVES, IEDS, BOOBY TRAPS, SUICIDE BOMBERS

"The God of peace is never glorified by human violence."
Thomas Merton

The first explosives are attributed to the Chinese, who mixed saltpeter, a common name for potassium nitrate, with sulfur and charcoal to form a powder which resulted in a burst of smoke and flames in the 9th century. [1]

"An Italian Chemist, Ascanio Sobrero (1812-1888), invented the first modern explosive Nitroglycerine, by treating glycerine with nitric and sulfuric acids in 1846". [2]

2. https://en.wikipedida.org>wiki>ascanio+Sobrero

"Dynamite is an explosive made of nitroglycerine sorbents (a material used to absorb or adsorb liquids or gases-https://en.wikipedia.org>wiki>Sorbent.), such as powdered shells or clay, and stabilizers [a chemical used to prevent degradation], was invented and patented by Alfred Nobel in 1867, in Geesthact, Northern Germany. He changed the name from Nobel's blasting powder to dynamite, from the Greek word meaning power". [dy]

It is reported that "After people foolishly misused his creation to kill, he regretted his invention". He died on December 10, 1896 and left his fortune of some 230 million dollars to start the Nobel Peace Prize Award.

Tri-nitrotoluene (TNT), is a second-generation castable explosive adopted by the military.

"Castable explosives, or castings are explosive materials or mixtures in which at least one component can be safely melted at a temperature which is safe to handle the other components, and which are normally produced by casting or pouring the molten mixture into a form or use container.

In modern usage TNT is the basic meltable explosive used in essentially all castable explosives.

More than 90% of the TNT produced in America was always for the Military.

Currently only Dyno Nobel manufactures dynamite in the United States, located in Carthage, Missouri".

In current terminology, a bomb may be a noun and a verb.

As a noun, "It is a fused explosive device designed to detonate under specified conditions (as impact). [3]

Another definition as a noun is "An explosive projectile originally consisting of a hollow ball or shell, filled with explosive materials, with a deep hollow sound", (possibly from the Latin Bombus, French Bombe or Greek Bombos); or, as in modern day football, a long bomb, a pass. [4]

As a verb it is 'painfully' seen in the constant bombing of Ukraine by Russia in daily news media reports. [3]

Bombs can be classified as conventional, as noted in Ukraine or atomic or thermonuclear. (See discussion in Chapter 7).

The explosive charge in conventional bombs may be TNT or ammonium nitrate.

They may also be "classified as to their use and the explosive material they contain; blast (demolition), fragmentation, general purpose, armor piercing, and incendiary (fire) bombs.

Demolition bombs destroy buildings or other structures where-as fragmentation bombs are lethal against personnel.

Incendiary bombs are of two main types, one using thermite, a mixture of aluminum powder and iron oxide against buildings and napalm, or jellied gasoline, against personnel.

Cluster bomb and fuel-air explosives ((FAE) where in dozens of small bomblets or an explosive vapor cloud explodes in the air, just above the ground, causing deaths or injuries. [cl]

Efforts to Ban the use of these weapons have been put forth by the Convention on Cluster Munitions in August 2010".

[cl] https://www.britannica.com/print/article/72491.

Explosions with blast injuries and their effects are classified in the following manner:

A. Primary-Direct blast, hollow viscus, ruptured ear drums injury.
B. Secondary-Most common injury, projectiles, penetrating.
C. Tertiary-Blunt trauma, head injuries, crush injuries,
D. Quaternary-Burn injuries, existing medical problems exacerbated.
E. Quinary-Chemical agents, dirty bomb (RDD), radiation. *

*https://www.ncbi.nim.nih.gov>books>NBK430914.

Recently, "Improvised Explosive Devices (IEDS) [i.e.] and Booby Traps have become weapons of War. [5]

These have been classified as a Package type of IED, Vehicle-Borne IEDS (VIEDs) and Suicide Bomb IED, all of which share a common set of components, an initiation system or fuse, an explosive fill, a detonator and a power supply for the detonator and a container. It is a *homemade* device causing death or injury, using chemicals, biological toxins or radiological materials.

Booby traps are designed to kill or incapacitate personnel, and are emplaced (hidden or buried) to improve effectiveness. Most are explosives and are victim activated but may be detonated remotely".

Suicide vests may be ladened with explosives or ball bearings sewn in its interior. [6]

[1] [i.e] http://globalsecurity.org/military/intro/ied.htm. clhttps://www.britannica. com(...)ChemicalProducts.

[2] https://en.wikipedia.org>wiki>Ascanio Sobrero.

[3] Webster All-In-One Dictionary & Thesaurus, Federal Street Press, 4th printing, 05/2010.

[4] dictionary.com/browse/bomb.

[5] https://counteriedreport.com>tags>suicide-vest.

[6] https://www.ciedcoe.org?repots-2016>file-

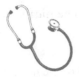

CHAPTER 9

FOREIGN AND DOMESTIC THREATS

Agro-terrorism
Demonic Terrorism

"While nothing is easier than to denounce the evildoer,
nothing is more difficult than to understand him"

Feodor Dostoyevsky [1]

Several definitions of Terrorism have been are presented in the Introduction. Common components noted in each of the definitions include criminal action, force or violence directed towards a civilian population for the purpose of advancing social or political objectives, with the intent of intimidating or coercing the population or the government. [2]

Domestic Terrorism has been the most common form of Terrorism in the United States (US); and prior to 9/11 the most deadly, in lives lost.

The Federal Bureau of Investigation (FBI) reported 353 incidents or suspected incidents in the US between 1980 and 2001, 264 all related to Domestic Terrorists. (1 p 114 Ibid) [3]

Further, in 2004 the FBI "stated Domestic Terrorisms are acts of violence that are violations of the criminal laws of the US by Groups without foreign direction, and appear to be intended to intimidate or coerce a civilian population or influence the policy of a government by intimidation or coercion and occurs primarily within the territorial jurisdiction of the United States. [4]

Domestic Terrorism is generally manifested in forms described as "left-wing, right-wing and special interest single issue Groups.

The Federal Bureau of Investigation (FBI) reportedly "prevented 10 possible terrorist events including two potentially large-scale high casualty attacks by right-wing groups." [5]

The Jewish Defense League which has committed attacks against the USA does not fit in either of the above groups.[6]

"George Metesky was described as a quiet man thus none of his neighbors suspected he was responsible for the bombing that terrorized New Yorkers for 16 years. In January 1952 he confessed to being *"the Mad Bomber"* who plotted 32 bombs in New York City injuring 16 people". [1, p118]

According to the Washington Post News Paper, June 11, 2023, Ted Kaczynski, "the Unabomber", a Harvard-trained mathematics prodigy who had killed three individuals whom he did not know with [series of pipe bombs], between 1978 to 1995, died in prison on June 10, 2023, cause of death yet to be determined.

Domestic *left-wing* philosophy seek to eliminate capitalism, over throwing or remaking the government, creating a society where all people are equal and prejudices do not exist, <u>with some form of</u> temporary government to ensure a smooth transition between capitalism and the ideal state. [6]

Examples of this Group were "the Weathermen, popular from 1969 to 1977, and "the Black Panther Party". [7]

Domestic *right-wing* philosophy is some-what the opposite of left-wing philosophy. Neo Nazi Groups which try to establish a strong military or nationalistic government is an example of this Group, as is the Klu Klux Klan (KKK).

The KKK developed in three distinct waves in the USA.

The first was in the Confederate States in the South in opposition to Reconstruction which threatened white supremacy. During this wave, many blacks were killed and Black Churches were destroyed.

The second wave, around 1915, was a response to the labor movement, when many Irish Catholics immigrated to the USA, following the *"potato blight"* in Ireland.

The third wave was in response to the civil rights movement and school integration.[6]

Some active special interests Groups are the Animal Rights, Anti-Abortion and the Environmental or Eco-terrorists. [6]

Cyber-terrorism of late has resulted in considerable financial disruption in the country.

The La Guardia Airport Bombing in 1975 with 11 killed, the World Trade Center in 1963 where 6 were killed and over 1,000 were injured and the Oklahoma City Bombing by Timothy McVeigh, where 168 were killed at the Murrah Federal Building were major incidents.

The most horrific Foreign Terroristic act was of course the 9/11 event in New York City where 2,977 were killed and over 6,000 injured.

[1] Sauter, Mark A., et al, Homeland Security-A Complete Guide to Understanding, Preventing and Surviving Terrorism. McGraw – Hill Chapter 4, p63, 2005

[2] Joint Publication DOD Dictionary__http//www.dtc.mie/doctrine/je1/doddist/.

[3] Federal Bureau of Investigation, Terrorism in the United States 1995 http//www.fbi.gov.

[4] www.fbi.gov/congress/congress04/lewis051805.htm

(Testimony of Robert S. Mueller III, Director FBI, February 11, 2003)

[5] www.fbi.gov/comgress03/mueller021103.htm.

[6] Instructor Guide, Train the Trainer, Terrorism Training, January 2004. Police 7 Correctional Training Commissions, 3085 Hernwood Rd, Woodstock Md., 21163-1099 Domestic Terrorist, p 5-24.

[7] Pearson, Hugh, The Shadow of the Black Panther, AddisonWesley Publishing Co., Reading Mass., 1994.

Lessons learned from the Oklahoma City bombing are reported in the Rand Study are noted in Chapter12, "The emotional and psychological effects on individuals who did not hear, see or feel the explosion". [8]

[8] The Milbank Quarterly, Vol 82 (3) 2004

Agroterrorism

The deliberate introduction of an animal or plant disease with the goal of undermining stability, causing economic losses and inducing fear in a population. The attacks could cause major economic crises in agricultural and food industries; also, human health would be at risk for possible transmission of diseases to humans (zoonosis).

The presence or rumor of certain animal or plant disease in a country can quickly stop exports of certain products, as was the case of beef from the United States of America (USA) to China in the Spring of 2008.

A major concern related to animal disease in the USA is the relatively limited experience of Veterinarians and Scientist with foreign animal disease.

Until 2006, according to the American Veterinary Medical Association, the number of Veterinarians from the 28 Veterinary Schools in the USA was approximately 2,700, with about 62,000 employed. That number was expected to increase by 35% by the end of 2006. *

Veterinarians work closely with the Public Health Department and in a Public Health emergency, they may be activated through State local systems such as the Emergency Support Functions (ESF) with the local Department of Health in Washington, DC, ESF #8. [1,2]

In 2022, there are approximately 48,000 Veterinarians in the USA, with an average annual salary of $123,000 dollars. [3]

Since the Anthrax event in this country in 2001, more attention has been focused on Veterinary Medicine, and more experience has been gained from working with some of the common diseases which affect farm animals, such as Foot and Mouth disease, E. coli, Influenza and Brucellosis and common animal pet diseases such as Hookworm, Ringworm, Roundworm, Salmonella, Psittacosis (Parrots Fever) and Lyme Disease. [4]

[1]Agroterrorism: Threats and Preparedness, updated, Feb., 2005,

Congressional Research Service [CRS]-the Library of Congress, Order code RL32391.

[2] Agricultural Bioterrorism: A Federal Strategy to Meet the Threat.
* http://www.ndu.edu/inss/ .
[3] https://vikaspedia.im>agriculture>livestocks>common-a.
[4] https://www.ucdavis.edu>one-health>most-common.

Cyberterrorism (CT)

The main types of Cyberterrorism attacks are Incursion, Destruction, Disinformation, Denial of services and Defacement of Web sites.

This Book will not attempt to present a discussion on this very dynamic topic, but lists a couple of sites from which pertinent information can be obtained.

(ct) https://resources.infosecinstitute.com>topic>spearphid...
https://us.cert.cisa.gov>ncas>alerts.

One area of significance we will note is Water Security.

The Environmental Protection Agency (EPA) has the responsibility to support disaster preparedness with tools that aid and design operation of

Water and Waste Water Systems in a way that decrease their vulnerability to disasters. (EPA).

Water Security-US EPA: https://www.epa.gov>emergemcy-response-research.

Demonic Terrorism

This is another form of Terrorism the author believes the reader should be aware of, constantly!

This form presents itself as Pride, Covetousness, Lust, Anger, Gluttony, Envy, Sloth and Gossip.

To counter these forms are the following Virtues: Humility, Liberality, Chastity, Meekness, Temperance, Brotherly Love, Diligence and not participating in Gossip. [9]

[8] Manual of Prayers, Pontifical North American College Rome, the Third Edition, p 48, nacrome @aol.com

CHAPTER 10

SPECIAL POPULATIONS

"The most pathetic person in the world is someone
who has sight, but has no vision".

Helen Keller

Pediatrics, Colleges, Universities, Dentistry, Group Homes, the
Intellectually Disabled, Nursing Homes, Prisons, Telehealth and Veterinary
Medicine

After a major disaster involving mass causality it is likely that Healthcare
Providers will treat victim of all ages. Mass causality exercises should
include victims of all ages, covering a range of mobility and possible
complications.

Pediatricians must be included in these exercises.

Pediatrics applies to infants and children from birth up to age 18, so
all health-related issues involved with this group is best addressed by
Pediatricians, Family Care Physicians and Specialists in this age group. [1]

Mental and emotional issues are always concerns of healthcare providers,
and significantly so in mass casualty disasters.

The Oklahoma bombing of the Federal Murrah Building in April, 1995 as reported in Table 3 of the Milbank Quarterly reports such effects on children. [2]

When the stories are written about the multiple killings of children by Russia in Ukraine, [3,4] up to this date, May7, 2022, one may be taken back to Biblical times when Herod had all the infant boys ages 2 years and younger, killed. [5]

With the exception of Vaccines for Covid-19 for children ages 5 to 11 years old, most Vaccines are an acceptable part of safe children's healthcare, and hopefully will not be a factor in addressing emergency preparedness in the Pediatric age group.

As of December 19, 2021, only the Pfizer-BioNTech Covid-19 Vaccine is authorized for children ages 5 through 17 years old. [6a,b,7]

By the time this book is published these recommendations may well have changed.

One specific Disease which has been noted as a result of the use of a Biological Weapon was the Botulinum Toxin, and has been associated with "infant botulism, when the bacterium Clostridium botulinum develops in the intestines and releases the toxin. This typically occurs in infants less than 6 months old and is associated with honey, which can contain the organism, so honey should not be fed to infants under 12 months old. Treatment is with an anti-toxin". [8]

As a result of the various natural disasters which have occurred involving earthquakes, hurricanes, tornadoes and wild fires, some 30 Colleges in the United States have developed Emergency Response Plans to address these issues. [9]

It is likely that most Physicians have, or should have an Emergency Response Plan in place, which all of the employees and Staff are thoroughly familiar with.

The state of preparedness of the facilities and the Healthcare providers, involved will serve to indicate what corrections, additions etc. are needed, such that when the actual disaster occurs all entities will be maximally prepared. *

*http://pediatrics.aappublications.org

Following by bombing of the Munich Federal Building in Oklahoma City, Oklahoma in 1995 and the destruction tornados in May 1999, the Emergency Medical Service Authority and Terrorism Research Center, founded in 1996 with worldwide networks in conjunction with Georgetown University, Biosecurity Institute, have prepared a document entitled Project Pediatric Preparedness, Final Report.

The report lays out in great detail fifteen functional areas for pediatric response including missions and tasks required for the emergency response, which this book does not list.

It is assumed that the Healthcare Providers recognize that as with any injury or illness involving a pediatric victim, the parents and/or responsible adults become a part of the management dynamic.

Project Pediatric Preparedness Final Report – unique requirements, goals, capabilities and gaps in Pediatric Preparedness and Response – Dr. Maria Powell, Mr. Neal A. Pollard, Esq., Mr. Kelly Deal – Terrorism Research Center, Inc., and Tulsa "Emergency Medical Service Authority" Grant Management Department, Tulsa OK.

With respect to biological agents, the signs and symptoms of exposure to certain agents, for example anthrax, plague and tularemia may be similar in adults and children; however, smaller concentrations and shorter exposure time to these agents are required for clinical manifestations. Children have a more rapid rate of respiration and smaller lung surface which translates into a higher degree of inhalation of area sized agents.

In the event of isolation or quarantine procedures involving Pediatric victims the psychological effects must be carefully planned for.

The American Academy of Pediatrics has prepared the Pediatric Disaster Preparedness Tool Kit which Pediatricians and Staff should be familiar with which can be retrieved at:

https://www.aap.org>patient-care-disasters-and-children.

Further, an update from the original Checklist of 2014, which should be a part of Hospital Administrators All Hazards Emergency Response Plan is available at:

https://emscimprovement.center>...ToolKits.

Important for the Pediatrician, and all healthcare providers, is the availability of the "211 Code", part of the 8 N11Codes of the North American Numbering Plan (NANP) discussed in Chapter 11.

The Healthcare provider should refer to local Public Health Department for guidance and assistance for all disaster situations.

1. www.cdc.gov/ncidad/hip/bio/13apr99APIC_cdcBioterrisim .PDF
2. Everett, WW, Coffin, SE, Strom BL, Acad. Emerg. Med; 2003 Tues; 10 (G):606-11.
3. Chung, Mandl, KD, Shannon M, Acad. Emerg Med. 2004 FEB 11 (20 – 143-8
4. The Washington post, April 9, 10 2022.
5. The New American Bible, 1989-1990 Edit., Matthew 2: 16-18.
[6a] https://www.fda.gov/media/150386/download
[6b] https://fdda.gov/meddia/144416/doc
[7] https://www.cdc.gov/hcp>imz>child-Adolescent.
[8] "Fact sheets-Botulism" (https//.who.int/news-room/fact-sheets/detail/botulism). WHO10 January 2018
[9] https/www.greatvaluecolleges.net>disaster-prepared...
[10] https://www.cdc.gov/cpr>readiness>longtermcare
[11] https://www.asp.org>patient-care-and-child

Dentistry

The following quote sums up what should be available at every Dental Facility, and Health care Providers facility also.

"Every Dental setting should have at least, a Basic Emergency Kit, that includes Oxygen, an automated External Defibrillator (AED), Albuterol (Rescue Inhaler), Aspirin, Diphenhydramine (Antihistamine), an Auto-injector of Epinephrine, Nitroglycerine, Glucose and a Fire Extinguisher". *

* http://decisionsindentistry.com>Articles.

Another report indicates that "over 60 % of emergencies seen by Dentists' is Syncope (fainting), with hyperventilation seen in 70%". **

**https://www.ncbi.nim.nih.gov>Articles?PMC1586863.

How To Improve Emergency Preparedness in Dental Offices, as reported in https://.mimic.com>dentists, suggests several action steps which are Creation of an Emergency Action Plan (EAP) and create a Business Continuity Plan.

According to the American Dental Association (ADA) other elements to be considered are equipment, personnel and back-up systems.

Guidance for help in developing an EAP is available at the CDC and by the Occupational and Safety Health Association (OSHA) in the following references. [1,2]

[1] https://www.cdc.gov>docs>emergact>emerg.
[2] Osha.gov/etools/evacuation-plans-procedures/eap.

The New York State Dental Association has a web site with up-to-date emergency response information at https://www.ada.org>research >oral-health-topics>m.

Nursing Homes

"According to data from the National Center for Health Statistics, as of 2016, in the United States (US) there were an estimated:

4,600 Adult Day service centers.

12,200 Home Health Agencies.

4,300 Hospices.

15,600 Nursing Homes.

28,900 Residential Care Communities". *

*health.usnews.com/health-news/best-nursing-homes/articles/nursing-homes-facts-and-statistics.

Norway and Switzerland are the top-ranking countries for providing care for the elderly.

https://lottie.org>care-guides>which-country-has-the -best-care-for-the-elderly.

The United States ranks 8th in the world for the wellbeing of the elderly.

https://www.washingtonpost.com>news>2013/10/03.

In the United States, Hanceville, Alabama, Tucson, Arizona and Mission Hills, California are cities with the number one rated Nursing Homes.

https://www.newsweek.com>Health>Stastistics.

Nursing Homes have been very much in the forefront in the past few years due to the large amount of covid-19 related deaths.

The total cases reported in the US as of May 11, 2022 was 80,065 and 992,377 deaths.

Usafacts.org/visualization/coronavirus-covid-19-spred-map/.

With respect to Emergency Management, the paradigm of Prevention, Preparedness, Response, Recovery and Mitigation, should be included in every Emergency Action Plan (EAP). (https://www.unr.edu>organizational-resilience-phase.

For additional assistance in preparing an EAP, the Nursing Home Incident Management System (NHICS) Guide Book, information is available at obtained at Emergency Prep @ahca.org.

Intellectual Disabilities

This is a particularly challenging Group to prepare an EAP for.

"The New York Disability and Health Program partnered with the Westchester Institute for Human Development to promote a multi-session program to train adults with Intellectual Disabilities to understand and be prepared for emergencies". *

*https://emergencygmanagement.byu.edu>emergency.PDF.

The Federal Emergency management Agency (FEMA) has a trove of Free Preparedness material regarding Disasters and Emergencies which can be accessed via Ready.gov/be-informed and Ready.gov/plan.

For children with Intellectual Disabilities, Fetal Alcohol Syndrome (FAS) and other Developmental Disabilities, information can be obtained at:

1-800-CDC-INFO/www.cdc.gov/ncbddd.
ww.cdc.gov/intellectualdisabilities.

Jails, Prisons

"There but for the grace of God, go I". *

John Bradford, 1553

There is a difference between a Jail and a Prison.

Jails are usually local facilities, under the jurisdiction of Cities, and are short-term facilities, in which individuals spend less than a year, while awaiting longer sentences if indicated.

Prisons are institutional facilities under control of the State or Federal government, in which offenders serve longer sentences. [2]

According to a document reported from the National Institute of Corrections (NIC) titled "Prisons and Disasters, Accession Numbers 021503,214, Prisons` are not prepared to respond to and recover from natural and man-made disasters". [1]

"Prisons and jails have already become major hotspots for coronavirus infection. [2]

More than 70,000 people have tested positive for the virus and more than 700 have died since march 2020".

The above quote is from the article "A Call for Effective Emergency Management of Correctional Facilities during Covid-19", by Akua Armstrong, Director, Criminal Justice Reform. (American progress. org/article/call-effective-emergency-management-correctional-facilities-covid-19). [3]

Ira P. Robbins reports on Lessons Learned from Hurricane Katrina in 2008, involving some 8,000 male and female inmates who had been evacuated. [4]

Irrespective of the institution of concern, at the time of the event, the 5 aspects of emergency management, Prevention, Preparedness, Response, Recovery and Mitigation, and the 4 phases of emergency management, Preparedness, Response, Recovery and Mitigation must be in play. [5]

*https://en.wikitionary.org>there-but-for-the-grace.
[1]. https://ncic.gov/prisons-and-disasters.
[2]. www.prisonfellowships.org/...faq-jail-prison.
[3]. https://americanprogress.org>article.call-effective-management-correctional-facilities-covid-19.
[4]. https://repository.law.umich.edu>mjer>vol42>iss.
[5]. https://training.fema.gov>emiweb>downloads/is111-unit%204.

Colleges, Universities, Schools

Following all of the events which have occurred in the country since the Oklahoma Bombing in April, 1995, by Timothy McVeigh, most academic institutions have in place, some form of Emergency Management Plan, as do many families.

At the K-12 level, one can find "School Emergency Preparedness: From The Inside Out" at https://www.ravemobilesafety.com>blog>k-12school.

Other references are ready.gov/kids/curriculum and https://www.dhs.gog>REMk-12Guide508_0. Guide for developing High Quality School Emergency Operation Plan.

https://www.depts.ttu.edu>k-12, from Texas Tech University.

An online academic program was established in the State of Texas in 1993.

Many Schools have in place now, Emergency Action Plans (EAP) in keeping with the most common disaster in the State, e.g., Earthquakes and Wild Fires, in California, Tornadoes in Oklahoma, and Hurricanes in Florida and communities along the Gulf Coast.

Telehealth

The article, "Telehealth in Emergency Preparedness and Response, defines Telehealth as the use of electronic information and telecommunication technologies to support healthcare delivery, health education, public health and health administration".

The article points out the "interaction of the emergency management cycle of preparedness, response, recovery and mitigation with virtual support, mobile alerts, the American Red Cross, and briefly describes the North American Treaty Organization (NATO), and the multi-national telemedicine systems that connect with Specialists located abroad". *

*https://healthcareready.org>uploads>2019/12>H.

Veterinary Medicine

The American Veterinary Medical Association, in an article, "Disaster Preparedness", presents information and tools on how to write a Disaster Plan for your Clinic.

More discussion regarding this area of medicine is noted earlier in the discussion on Agroterrorism in Chapter 9.

ava.org/resources-tools/animal-health-and-welfaee/disaster-prepaedness.

Emergency planning information for Veterinary practices is also available at:

https://www.avma.org>disaster-prepaedness-emergency.

CHAPTER 11

CURRENT STATE OF PREPAREDNESS

"Never let your sense of morals prevent you from doing what is right".

Isaac Asimov

When approaching any disaster, the Healthcare provider should keep in mind the Emergency Management Cycle, which includes the following phases: Preparedness, Response, Recovery and Mitigation. [1]

Basic Life Support (BLS)

Heimlich maneuver
Abdominal thrust
Chest thrust

Every Healthcare Provider should be prepared to provide Basic Life Support, and ideally, Advance Life Support, if needed. (aha)

In the presence of a witnessed or suspected heart attack in an adult or child, the first 10 seconds are critical.

During this time, an assessment of the situation should be done by seeing if the individual is conscious and responding, checking to see if the individual is breathing properly, checking for a pulse, and call 911, or asking a bystander, if present, to do so.

Further, many individuals wear necklaces or bracelets indicating certain illness they have.

Many individuals now have Cell Phones.

If this situation occurs in an adult, consideration of a heart attack must be a priority, and according to current concepts advanced by the American Heart Association (AHA), "The Adult Chain of Survival" should be introduced.

This consists of:

1. "Immediate recognition of cardiac arrest and activation of the emergency response system.
2. Early cardiopulmonary resuscitation (CPR) with emphasis on chest compression.
3. Rapid defibrillation.
4. Effective advanced life support.
5. Integrated post-cardiac arrest care".

"In children the cardiac arrest may be secondary to respiratory failure or shock".

In each event, "chest compression should be started within 10 seconds of recognition of a cardiac arrest. In adults and children, compression at the lower end of the sternum, using both hands should be hard and fast for 100 compression per minute, with a depth of at least 2 inches, (5 cm), and approximately 1 ½ inches (4cm) in infants.

For all ages, (except for newborns), begin CPR with compression (C-A-B sequence). After each set of chest compressions, open the airway and give 2 breaths."

"The 2010 AHA Guidelines for CPR and emergency cardiovascular care recommend a change in the BLS sequence of steps from A-B-C (Airway, Breathing, Chest compression) to C-A-B (Chest compression, Airway, Breathing) for adults, children and infants."

(aha) American Heart Association, BLS for Healthcare Providers Student manual, 20011, ISBN 978-1-61689-039-7.

If an Automated External Defibrillator (AED) is available, it should be employed as soon as possible for adults and children 8 years of age and older. (aha, part 3)

The Author strongly recommends that the reader makes contact with their local Chapter of the American Heart Association and/or the American Red Cross, for training and updates on these measures.

Other skills which the healthcare provider should be familiar with are the Heimlich maneuver, abdominal thrusts and chest thrusts.

The Heimlich maneuver was invented by Dr. Henry Heimlich (1920-2016), a Jewish American Thoracic Surgeon in 1974. (hm).

Initially the maneuver employed the use of 5 sharp blows to the back of an individual suspected of "choking", after having asked him/her to try and cough.

It is reported that Heimlich himself asked that the phrase "Heimlich maneuver" be removed from the literature and replaced with the phrase *"abdominal thrust"*, because he wanted the back blows stopped.

In unconscious individuals, 1 year old and older, this technique is still used.

The "chest thrust" [ct] is performed by "placing a clinched fist above the navel, the lower rib cage, then grasping the fist with the other hand, then pulling the clinched fist sharply, directly upward and backward under the rib cage 5 times quickly...may be used for obese persons and pregnant females".

(1) https://www.st.louis-mo.gov>public- safety>about>Step
(2) https://www.urmc.rochester.edu>Encyclopedia

"Choking-adults or children over 1 year/" Medline Place, NIH.

The following links can be viewed for a demonstration of the maneuver:

(hh) http://www.wikihow.com /Perform-the-Heimlich-maneuver.
(hh) https://en.wikipedia.org>wiki>Henry Heimlich.

He also invented the Heimlich Valve which allows air and blood to drain from the chest cavity to allow a collapsed lung to re-expand.

In 2006, Guidelines of the AHA and American Red Cross, replaced the term Heimlich maneuver with "abdominal thrusts", or if necessary "chest thrusts".

"Part 5, Adult Basic Life Support and Cardiopulmonary Quality, emergency care (EC) Guidelines".

ct ecguidelines.heart.org.

In 2002, Congress passed the Public Health Security and Bioterrorism Act for approximately $11 Billion annually for states to strengthen public health preparedness. Billions more were invested and there is yet incomplete state-by-state readiness information.

Beginning in 2003 and annual issue report titled "Ready or Not: Protecting the Public's Health from Diseases, Disaster and Bioterrorism", prepared by Trust for American Health (TFAH) was released.

Former General Lowell Weicker Jr. was the President of the Board of Director. The Report was prepared by some 24 individuals representing public and private interests.

Using 10 indicators applied to each state and the District of Columbia. Among the conclusions were:

1. Five years after 9/11 Public Health Emergency was still not at acceptable level.

2. Although limited progress has been made the over achieving goals of adequate preparedness remain unmet

3. American citizens continue to face unnecessary and unacceptable high levels of risks Diseases, Disasters and Bioterrorism.

As of December 2006, the indicators revealed the following findings:

Strategic National Stockpile (SNS), only 14 states and 2 cities were rated at the highest level of preparedness (New York and Chicago were the two cities) for providing emergency vaccine, antidotes, and medical supplies for the SNS.

Bio-Threat Testing, eleven states and DC did not have adequate capabilities to test for biological threats.

Trained Laboratory Scientists; four states lacked adequate lab experts trained to test for outbreak of anthrax or plague.

Pandemic Flu Surveillance – year-round Influenza testing – four states did not test on a year-round basis, necessary for monitoring a Pandemic Flu Outbreak

Hospital Bed Surge Capacity for Pandemic Flu- half of the states were have no hospital beds left within 2 weeks of a moderately severe pandemic flu outbreak.

Seasonal Flu Vaccinations – influenza vaccinations decreased for serious in 13 states.

Pneumonia Vaccinations – the National median for pneumonia vaccination in seniors is 65.7%. The National goal for 2010 is 90%.

National Electronic Disease Surveillance – twelve states are not fully compatible with the CDC's National

Electronic Surveillance System (NEDSS) to track outbreak information.

Nursing Shortage – Forty States and the District of Columbia have a shortage of Registered Nurses.

Public Health Budgets – six states had Public Health Budgets cut between 2004 -2005 and FY 2005-2006. As of FY 2005-2006 the median state funding for public health was $31 per person per year.

All of the above information may well have changed since this initial writing, especially following the Covid-19 pandemic of 2020.

For viewing your states or city's level of readiness and much more detail go the www.HealthAmerican.org, Trust for America's Health, 2006.

A similar report was completed in 2007 which did show overall improvements.

In February 2008 the CDC published key findings from Public Health Preparedness; mobilizing state-by-stat, reporting on nine preparedness goals, similar to the 10 indicators reported on by TFAH – The number of Epidemiologists and Public Health laboratories have increased, was a part of the Laboratory Response Network – All states can now receive supplies from the SNS in 12-hours or less, as well as store and distribute them; all states and DC now participate in the Health Alert Network (HAN) communication system allowing for raped exchange of critical public health information. A secure CDC-based Communication System the Epidemic Information Exchange (EPI-X) that helps track disease outbreaks as significantly increased to 4,646 in 2006 up from 890 in 2001.

Challenges remain in the area of work force recruiting and retaining qualified Public Health Scientists, Nurses and Physician in the Medical and Nurses Reserve Corp. Rapid identification of radioactive material remains a problem.

Although there has been increased training in risk communication and mental health, there remains legal issues, addressing at risk populations, the Pediatric population and the issue of quarantine and isolation

There remains the need for expanding interoperable communications across jurisdictions and various levels of government.

More information on current state of preparedness and how to prepare for an emergency can be found at:

http://emergency.cdc.gov, www.nphic.ore/regions.asp,vers: Mobilizing state-by-state go to: http://emergency.cdc/gov/publications/feb08phpre for the full report on Public Health Prepared by the CDC.

Strategic National Stockpile (SNS).

The Strategic National Stockpile is the nation's largest supply of medical countermeasures for use in a public health emergency, severe enough to cause local supplies to be depleted.

"The Public Health Service Act #319F-2;42U.S.C.#247d-6b authorizes the secretary of Health and Human Services, in coordination with the secretary of Homeland Security, to maintain a stockpile of drugs, vaccines and other medical products and supplies, known as the Strategic National Stockpile (SNS) to provide for the emergency health security of the United States and its territories.

State Governors or their designees, or the Mayor of Washington, DC, may request deployments of SNS assets and a {Push Package}, caches of medicines and medical supplies can be delivered to the requesting entity within 12 hours, less in Washington, DC". *,**

For a detailed account of the SNS see:

*www.cdc.gov/phpr/stockpile/stockpile.htm,　　also,　　**https://www.astho.org/Programs/Prepardness/Public-Health-Emergency-Law/Emergency-Use-authorization-Toolkit/Strategic-National-Stockpile-Fact-...

Components of the SNS include the following:

"CHEMPACKS, containers of Nerve Agent Antidotes placed in secure locations in local jurisdictions around the country to allow rapid response to a chemical incident. These medications treat the symptoms of nerve agent exposure and can be used even when the actual agent is unknown". https://www.phe.gov>aboutSNS>Pages>CHEMPAC.

A CHEMPACK Hospital Formulary may include Mark-I, II Kits, Atropine Sulfate 0.4 mg/ml, Diazepam 5 mg/ml auto-injector, Pralidoxime 1 gm injector, 20 ml (2-PAM) and Diazepam 5 mg/ml vial.

Chemm.hhs.gov/antidote_nerveagents.htm.
http://www.heath.ny.gov>emspdf.

Cities Readiness Initiative (CRI) "is a federally funded program, designed to enhance preparedness in the nation's largest population centers where nearly 60% of the population resides, to effectively respond to large public health emergencies needing life-saving medicines and medical supplies.

As of November 2019, the CRI project began in 2004 with 21 cities and has expanded to include a total of 72 cities and metropolitan statistical areas (MSAs) with at least one CRI city in every state". https://www.cdc.gov/cpr/readiness/mcm/cri.html.

Another entity involved in this process is "The Global Health Security Agenda (GHSA), a partnership U.S. government sister agencies, other nations, international organizations and public and private stakeholders. The program seeks to accelerate progress towards a world safe and secure from infectious disease threats and to promote global health security as an international security priority, to prevent, detect and respond to public health threats within their borders". https:/www.phe.gov/about/sns/Pages/global.aspx.

To fund these programs is "The Public Health Emergency Preparedness (PHEP) cooperative agreement [2019-2024], a critical source of funding for state, local and territorial departments". https://.www.cdc.gov/cpr/readiness/phep.htm.

Evacuation

Since the events of 911 and the Anthrax deaths in Washington, DC in 2001, disaster planning has been in the forefront in many Public Health and private facilities. These Plans include an All-Hazards Response at local, state and territorial levels and a process for evacuations.

According to the reference listed below, there are 4 types of evacuations:

1. Stay (Shelter) in place; when a biological or chemical event is suspected.
2. Building evacuation.
3. Campus evacuation
4. City evacuation

https://www.ready.gov>evacuation.

Every family should have a Family Disaster/Evacuation Plan with a "Go Bag" at the ready. Ideally food, water and critical medicines should be in the bag, enough for 3-7 days.

Be sure that more than one person is involved in the planning, especially for any disabled family members.

For assistance in this category see http://www.redcross.org/get-help/how-to-prepare-for-emergencies/disaster-safety-for-people-with-dissabilities#Plan-Ahead.

Any Plan must include pets, with their own "Go Bag". Further, a collar or harness, a leash, a crate or pet carrier, as well as an ID tag with Rabies information should be included.

Some important references for assistance with this preparation are:

https://www.redcross..org>get-help>make-a-Plan
https://www.osha.gov>emergency-preparation>get.
https://www.fema.gov>site.default>file>pla.PDF.
https://www.disastercenter.com?guide>family.
https://www.ready.gov/pet-toolkit.
https://www.ready.gov/animals.

Medical Surge.

    A. Surge Capacity
    B. Surge Capability

In major disasters, health care departments must be prepared to handle mass casualty incidents (MCI) and mass effect incidents (MEI). [1]

Mass casualty incidents are defined as "those in which emergency medical services resources, such as personnel and equipment are overwhelmed by the number and severity of casualties".

In the pre-hospital phase of a mass casualty response, assuring the safety of responders, before casualties, should be a primary feature.

Among the myriad responses for a successful outcome, an essential response must be strict scene and hospital security.

[1,2]https://en.wikipedia.org>wiki>Mass- casualty incident.

Mass effect incident is "an incident that primarily affects the ability of the organization to continue normal operations".

[1,2]https://www.phe.gov/Preparedness/planning/mscc/handbook/chapter1.

"Medical *surge* describes the ability to provide adequate medical evaluation and care during events that exceed the limits of the normal medical infrastructure of an affected community.

In order to respond appropriately, there is a need to distinguish between surge capacity and surge capability.

Medical surge *capacity* refers to the ability to respond to an increase volume of patients with an adequate number of hospital beds, personnel, medical supplies and equipment. In order that this works well, appropriate systems and process must be in place that in fluence specific asset quantity.

Medical surge *capability* refers to the ability to manage patients requiring unusual or specialized evaluation and care".

Lessons learned from previous mass casualty incidents has resulted in the need for and establishing of mutual aid systems.

Mutual *aid* "involves sharing resources and services between jurisdictions and organizations. This assistance can include the daily dispatch of law enforcement, emergency medical and fire services resources between local communications, as well as movement within a state or across state lines.

Mutual Aid agreements establish the legal basis for two or more entities to share resources."

Within the United States this process is guided through a congressionally ratified mutual aid compact called the Emergency Management Assistance Compact (EMAC).
(https://emac.org) en.wikipedia.org/wiki/Mutual_aid_(Organization_Theory)

Numbering Resources

9 N11 Codes of North American Plan (NANP) *

"Effective February 9, 2021, the Federal Communication Commission (FCC) **granted petitions filed by the US Department of Transportation (DOT), and by Information and Referral providers seeking nationwide assignment of abbreviated dialing Codes, or use of the N11codes and other abbreviated assignments.

Some of these Codes are:

211 Essential Community Services.

311 Non-emergency Police and Governmental

Services.

711 A telephone service that allows persons with hearing or speech disabilities to receive and place calls.

911 The 911 Act as of October 1999, makes 911 the universal emergency number for all telephone calls.

988 Suicide hot line added in July 2022.

*https//en/Wikipedia.org>wiki>N11_codes.
**https://doc.fcc.gov>public>attachments.   DOC-358075A2.pdf-Federal Communications Commission.

Quarantine/Isolation

"The good of the people is the chief law"

Cicero-,106-43- BC.

According to the Oxford Dictionary, Quarantine is a period of isolation imposed a person, animal or thing that might other-wise spread a contagious disease.

Isolation is the separation of individuals known or suspected, via signs, symptoms, laboratory criteria or recent trave, to be infected with a contagious disease to prevent transmission to others.

The word Quarantine comes from word *quaresma,* which means 40, in Italian *quaranta giorni.* This refers to the 40 days of sequestration imposed on arriving ships from Venice during the Plague outbreak, *the Black Death,* in 1938.) [bd]

[bd]htpp://72.14.290.104/search?q=cache:megUlqvT6QJ:en.wikipedia.org.org/wiki/Quarantine+qu.

In 1893 the United States (US) Congress passed the National Quarantine Act and in 1949, the Public Health Services Act was codified, establishing quarantine authority with the Federal government which has controlled all quarantine stations since 1921. [qs]

[qs] http://www.cdc.govncidod/dq/quarantine_stations.htm.

In 1967 responsibility was transferred to the National Communicable Disease Center, now the Center for Disease Control and Prevention (CDC).

In April 2003, the revised list of Quarantinable Communicable Diseases, by the President's Executive Order #13295, section 361(b) of the Public Health Services Act, are noted below.

As President Biden contemplates mandating vaccination in order to combat Covid, it is important to reflect on previous attempts at mandates, and unintended consequences.

In 1893, an outbreak of Small pox in Muncie, Indiana [mi] resulted in entire neighborhoods being quarantined and the area patrolled with guards in place, with violators being arrested.

Mandatory vaccinations were instituted. Violence broke out and many civilians and public health officials were shot.

Later public health officials concluded that their efforts had failed.

(mi) Bioterriorism, Guidelines for Medical and Public Health Management, edited by Henderson, DA, Inglesby,TV, O'Toole, Journal of the American Medical Association (JAMA), 2002, p224-225.

Currently there are 20 Quarantine stations in the United States at Ports of Entry, Borders where international passengers can be screened and legally restrained if indicated.

https://www.hsdl.org>abstract.

In the midst of the severe acute respiratory syndrome (SARS) event, on April 4, 2003 President George W. Bush signed Executive Order 13295, issuing a revised list of quarantinable diseases, eight specific diseases, adding to the list SARS. In 2005, the Order was amended to include Influenza caused by novel remerging influenza viruses. ᵉᵒ

The current diseases are Cholera, Diphtheria, Infectious Tuberculosis, Plague, Small pox, Yellow Fever, the Viral Hemorrhagic Fevers, including Ebola, Lassa, Marburg, Crimean-Congo, Influenza, SARS and Measles. (qds)

Covid-19 and its variants will likely be added to the list.

(eo) http://influenzapreparedness.blogspot/
(qds) https://www.hhs.gov.answers>public_health_and-safety.
https://www.hhs.gov>answers>public-health-and-safety.

The initial response to a disaster should be a *situational awareness* of the event or Threat Assessment.

The 5 "Ws" are one approach to this issue which are:

1. What is it?
2. Where is it?
3. When was it?
4. Why is it there?
5. Whether anything? (Is it a Hoax)?

https://en.wikipedia.org/wiki/Five W.

Another version reflects the addition of the letter "H", which stands for "How or How Much"

https://www.guora.com>what-are-the-5 Ws and H-in.
https://K12.thoughtfullearning.com>minilesson>asking.

Start

The Simple Triage and Rapid Transport (START) method was developed in 1988 by staff members of the Hoag Hospital and Newport Beach Fire Department in California.

http://www.ncbi.nim.nih.gov/Articles>PMC5649292.
https://en.wikipedida.org>wiki>Simple-triage-and-rapid...

In healthcare, Triage is "the grouping of patients based on the severity of their injuries, and the likely-hood of their survival".

https://www.Sciencedirect.com>medicine and disast er.

It is based on the assessment of 3 criteria: Respirations, Perfusion and Mental status in 30 seconds.

These concepts will be in play with local departments of Health in disaster events.

"It's A Disaster!..and what are you gonna do about it?

A Disaster Preparedness, Prevention and First Aid Manual from the District of Columbia Homeland Security and Emergency Management Agency, 5th Edition, 2009, is available at:

www.itsadisaster.net or call at 1-888-999-4325.

This book may have been updated but it contains valuable information on all kinds of disasters.

Vaccines

"With the exception of water, no other modality, not even antibiotics, has had such a major effect on mortality reduction", according to (Platkins, S., Orenstein, W., Offit, P., Vaccines, 5th Ed., Saunders 2008).

Much of the following is extracted from an article entitled "Vaccines: How and Why", by Okenek and Peters in the Access Excellence Classic Collection, September 2005. [1]

http://www.accessexcellence.org/AE/AEC/CC/vaccines_how_why.htm[1]

"In the early1700s it was observed that some individuals infected with Small Pox, a disease characterized by pus filled blisters, starting on the face, mouth and hands, if the recovered, appeared not to be symptomatic if exposed to the disease.

The Chinese, in an attempt to prevent Small Pox, having observed this phenomenon used some of the pus and fluid from an infected person and placed in under the skin of an uninfected person, using a needle, a process called *'Variolation.'*

Another method was to use some of the peeling scabs which form in about 17 days, drying it and making it into a fine powder and letting the uninfected person inhale it.

Yet another method was to place a small amount of the *'scab powder'* on a needle and injecting it into the uninfected person's vein.

This latter method was reportedly observed by 'Lady Mary Wortles Montague', the wife of the British Ambassador to Turkey and brought back to England. There were some deaths associated with these techniques but overall, the mortality and morbidity appeared to be lower from Small Pox in those individuals so 'Variolated'."

"In the late 1700 a child by the name of Edward Jenner in England was 'Variolated' and survived after being infected with Small Pox. Jenner became a Country Doctor in England and noted that there was a relationship between Equine disease in horses known as 'Grease' and a Bovine disease in cows called 'Cow Pox'. He noted that farmers' who treated their horses with material from grease lesions, often saw development of Cow Pox in their cows with blisters similar to Small Pox, however these blisters disappeared and the disease was not lethal. He further noted that a Milk

Maid had told him that she could not catch Small Pox because she had Cow Pox, and there were many workers who milked cows and did not get Small Pox, although repeatedly exposed.

In 1776 he infected a young boy with Cow Pox with the intent of preventing Small Pox. After the boy fully recovered from Cow Pox, he injected pus from a Small Pox lesion in the boy's skin.

The boy did not contract Small Pox as Jenner predicted.

Jenner collected 23 cases and published his observations with the result that within a few years, thousands of people were protecting themselves against Small Pox by initially becoming infected with Cow Pox.

Later the process became known as *'Vaccination'*.

The word 'vacca' is Latin for cow and the substance use called *'vaccine'*.

The effect of the vaccine is to induce an immune response in the infected individual (Host). Antibodies are formed and Memory Cells are produced which may remain for the life time of the Host". (This process is via humoral immunity, to be discussed later).

"There are several ways to make Vaccines. One way is to kill the organism using Formalin. These Vaccines are called inactivated or killed Vaccines.

Examples of this type are the Typhoid Vaccine and the Salk Poliomyelitis Vaccine.

Another method is to use the antigenic part of the disease-causing organism e.g., the capsule or flagella or part of the protein wall. These are called Acellular Vaccines. An example of this is the Hemophilus Influenza B (HIB) Vaccine. (Antigen, defined later).

Both killed and Acellular Vaccines require a 'booster' every few years to continue the effectiveness. These are considered safe for use in immune compromised individuals.

Another method is to *'attenuate or weaken'* a live microorganism by aging or altering the growth patterns. These are often the most successful vaccines causing a large immune response; however, they can mutate back to the virulent form, and as such are not recommended for immune compromised individuals.

Examples of Attenuated vaccines are those against Mumps, Measles and Rubella (MMR). In most instances immunity is lifelong and 'booster shots' are not required.

Vaccines may also be made from Toxins. The Toxin may be treated with aluminum or adsorbed onto the aluminum salt to lessen its harmful effects; such vaccines being called *'Toxoids'*.

Examples of these are the Diphtheria and Tetanus vaccines. Because these vaccines may induce low level responses they are sometimes administered with an *'adjuvant'*, or an agent which increases the response.

The classic type of this vaccine is the DPT with Pertussis, the agent causing 'Whooping Cough' acting as the adjuvant.

Toxoid vaccines generally require a booster every 10 years.

Currently a common example of combining a virulent microorganism with a relatively mild organism, similar to Jenner's use of Cow Pox and Small Pox, is the Bacillus Calmette Guerin (BCG), used to protect against Tuberculosis. The BCG vaccine uses the attenuated strain of Mycobacterium bovis and the individual must have a booster every 3-4 years".

Allbert Calmette, a Physician and his colleague Camile Guerin a Veterinarian, developed the strains in the early 1900s. The vaccine was first used in humans in1921, given to a child in Paris France whose mother had died of Tuberculosis.

(Calmette, A, "Preventive vaccination against tuberculosis with BCG", Proc Roy Med, 1931:2485-94 *www.ncib.nlm.nih.gov/pmc/articles/PMC2/).

"Genetic Engineering techniques are used to produce *'subunit vaccines'*, vaccines which use only parts of an organism which stimulates a strong immune response. These are formed by a process called 'transcribing'. Hepatitis B vaccine is an example of these vaccines and is safe for use in immune compromised individuals because they do not cause the disease."

Vaccines play a positive role in protecting individuals as well as communities.

This type of community protection, referred to as *'Herd Immunity'*, works by decreasing the number of susceptible individuals. The greater the number of vaccinated individuals in a community the more rapidly will the disease disappear, due to the decreasing number of susceptible people". **

**http://www.accesseyexcellence.org/AE/AEC/cc/vaccines_home_why.html

These processes commonly occur in the Influenza viruses A, B and C by an Antigenic drift, where by two or more different strains or strains of two or more different viruses combine to form a new subtype.

Antigenic shift occurs only in Influenza A, because it infects more than humans. Influenza B and C infect humans primarily.

Antigenic shift is a major change in the Influenza A virus and most people do not have immunity to the novel, new subtype.

Antigenic drift and shift were earlier discussed in Chapter 4 with Influenza.

"Problems which may occur with use of viruses as vaccines include sensitization, reversion and possible complications.

Attenuated vaccine s should not be given to pregnant or immune compromised individuals. Another common problem includes the multiple serotypes of viruses and the processes of Antigenic drift and shift.

In the future, Genetic Engineered DNA vaccines, along with synthetic peptides and improved adjuvants, liposomes and saponin complexes will be part of the tool box". ***

***http://www.microbiologybytes.com/virology/vaccines.html

With respect to the Influenza flu shots and the recent H_1N_1 influenza shots, these are recommended.

Questions may arise for individuals who have cancer and their caregivers. *[1]

These individuals should be vaccinated. If one is to begin Chemotherapy, the flu shot can be taken before starting it or if chemo has been started the shot can be given a day or two before the next treatment begins.

If Radiation therapy is indicated, the shot can be given at any time *[2]

Tamiflu, the antiviral drug may be effective in cancer patients but it should be discussed with the Oncologist as it should be started within 48 hours of developing symptoms. *[2]

[1] www.health.gov.on.ca/en/ccom/flu/h1n1/publis/
[2] www.sdhu.com/index.asp?lang=0

"One of the adjuvants added to vaccines is Squalene, which is a naturally occurring substance found in plants, animals and humans. In humans it is manufactured in the liver and is commercially extracted from fish oil, Shark oil primarily." *[3]

Twenty- two million doses of Chiron`s Influenza vaccine (FLUAD0 have been administered since 1997. The vaccine contains about 10mgms of Squalene per dose and as of 2009, no severe adverse events have been associated with the vaccine". *[3]

[3] "http://www.who.int/vaccinein%20safety/topics/adjuvants/squalene/questions_and_answers/en/"

The following can serve as a useful review:

"The types of vaccines are: *[4]

Immunologists Tool box Appendix pp683-719, Immunobiology 6th Ed, 2005, Janeway, Travers, Garland, Science New York & London ISBN 0-8253-4101-6.

Live attenuated (weakened).

Inactivated (killed).

Toxoids (inactivated toxins).

Subunit (antigenic fragments).

Conjugates (to increase immune stimulation, used for young children who don't generate a strong immune response).

The principal vaccines used in the United States to prevent Bacterial Disease are:

Diphtheria (Toxoid)

Meningococcus meningitis

Pertussis

Pneumococcal pneumonia

Tetanus

Hemophilus meningitis

The principal vaccines currently used to prevent Viral Diseases are:

Influenza

Measles/Mumps/Rubella (MMR).

Chicken Pox

Small Pox

Poliomyelitis

Rabies

Hepatitis B

With the advent of covid-19 and Monkey pox, vaccines have been developed against these diseases, and newer vaccines have been developed for Ebola, covid-19 and Respiratory Syncytial virus (RSV).

There likely are other vaccines that are not included in this Book and searches with the WHO and CDC should be made for those, given the emerging infectious diseases occurring around the world.

Principal vaccines being developed against Bio-threats or new agents: include:

Bacillus anthracis (Anthrax).
Yersinia pestis (Plague).
Francisella tularensis (Tularemia).
Botulinum toxin (Botulism).
West Nile Virus.
Severe Acute Respiratory Syndrome (SARS).
Ebola (vaccine available in 2018, see discussion on Ebola).

Examples of live attenuated bacterial vaccines:

Typhoid (new oral vaccine).
Tuberculosis (TB) Bacillus Calmette-Guerin [BCG].
Meningitis
Mycobacterium bovis.
Salmonella?

Advantages and disadvantages of live attenuated viruses:

PROS:

May replicate in the body providing a strong immune response, including T cells and CD (CD 4 helper, CD8 cytotoxic) cells.
May require booster injections.
May provide long term protection, often life time.
High rate of success (often 95 %).

CONS:

May mutate to a virulent form.
Not recommended for immune compromised patients.

"Examples of Inactivated (killed) vaccines": [4]

Poliomyelitis (Salk)
Influenza
Rabies
Pneumococcal pneumonia
Cholera
Pertussis (Whooping cough)
Typhoid (old vaccine being replaced by attenuated form).

"Advantages and Disadvantages": [4]

Inactivated (Killed) vaccines cannot replicate in the body, therefore are safe for the immune compromised patients.

Provide a relatively weak immune status.
Do not stimulate CD 4 or 8 & T cells.
"Examples of Toxoid Vaccines (inactivated toxins)". [4]
Tetanus, Diphtheria

"Advantages and Disadvantages of Toxoid Vaccines": [4]

Do not replicate in the body, therefore are safe for immune compromised patients.
Directly blocks the toxic effects of the organism.
Requires a series of injections for full immunity, followed by boosters every 10 years.
Subunit Vaccines.

Recombinant proteins:

Recombinant refers to a cell or organism whose genetic material results from combining segments of DNA from different sources. (The Free Dictionary by Farlex).

"An alternative application of recombinant DNA technology is the production of Hybrid virus vaccines. These are relatively cheap and easy to produce and are stable and stimulate both cellular and humoral immunity". [4]

Cellular immunity uses T (Thymus) Cells to tag and destroy foreign antigens.

(c,h). https://www.reference.com/science/difference-between-cellular-humoral-immunity-cf93468a67329b).

Antigen- any substance that causes the immune system to produce antibodies against it.

(medlineplus.gov/ency/article/002224.htm).

Humoral immunity uses B cells or antibodies in the blood serum which attaches to the antigen, kills it/them and differentiates to form memory cells, specific for each antigen (c,h).

Rabies vaccine for animals and experimental HIV and Dengue vaccines are noted.

(Different Types of Vaccine, Live Attenuated Vaccines, DNA Vaccine... http://74.125.93.132/search?q=cache:W2yZEWkZrHwJ:virology-onli)

Produced by Genetic Engineering, e.g., hepatitis B surface antigen (HbsAg).

Synthetic peptides from individual proteins.

Conjugated Vaccines:

Used for young children who do not generate a strong immune response to certain antigens.

Combine polysaccharides with strongly immunogenic proteins; e.g., Diphtheria, Toxoid, Hemophilus influenza Vaccines.

Another concept of immunization is *Ring Vaccination* by which all susceptible individuals in a prescribed area around an outbreak of an infectious disease is immunized. (Previously discussed).

DNA vaccines are still under development and currently being used in clinical trials for Malaria and HIV." [*4]

An excellent overview of Immunizations is presented in: [Iz]

[Iz] About.com:Health-Topics, AZ http://adam.about.com/reports 000090 2.htl

In 2021, reports from https://www.npace.org and https:///www.cdc.gov>hpv>parent>vaccine-for-hpv, recommended vaccination for the Human Papilloma Virus (HPV) starting at ages 11 to 12 years old for males and females, for the prevention of certain cancers.

Consultation with a Pediatrician is strongly recommended.

Clinical Trials.

Before new drugs or vaccines are approved for use in the USA they are subjected to the Investigational New Drug (IND) [*5] process, designed to allow individuals or any academic institution, Drug Company or any other Organization to bring a product to market for public use.

Once the product is considered safe for human use, data as to the risks of use are then obtained by early-stage Clinical Trials

The IND is not an application for marketing approval and applies to investigators and sponsors.

The types of INDs are Investigators, Emergency use and Treatment. Emergency Use and Treatment are also known as Compassionate INDs

There are two categories, Commercial and Non-commercial (Research).

There are three Phases of investigation and an IND may be submitted for one or more Phases.

Phase I is the initial study, usually with between 20-80 healthy volunteers. The mechanisms of action side effects and measures of effectiveness are recorded in this Phase.

Phase II involves several hundred people with a known condition or disease to obtain data and effectiveness and any side effects and risks.

Phase III gathers further information on effectiveness in order to evaluate the overall benefit-risk relationship of the product.

This Phase involves several hundred to several thousand individuals, allowing for extrapolating results to the general public, and transmitting it in the Physician Labeling Formulary.

[*5] http://www.fda.gov/cder/about/smallhiz/fag.htm .

The status of new vaccines is reported by the Centers for Disease and Prevention (CDC), weekly/October 212016/65 (45); 1136-1140.

The report notes, "Historically, new vaccines only became available in low income and middle-income countries decades after being introduced in high income countries. The Pneumococcal Conjugate Vaccine (PCV), the Roto Virus for infants and the Human Papilloma Virus (HPV) are examples of vaccines available worldwide."

New and improved vaccines for diseases such as Meningitis, Cholera, Typhoid, Ebola (in 2018), Dengue and Zika are now available, or likely to be, by the time this book is published.

According to the World Health Organization (WHO)* "The wide spread use of RTS, S/AS01 (RTS) Malaria vaccine is recommended among children in sub-Saharan Arica and in other regions with moderate to high P. falciparum malaria transmission".

*https://www.int>News>item.

Also new are the Johnson and Johnson, Moderna and Pfizer vaccines for covid-19 developed in 2020.

A more detailed discussion of these vaccines is in the discussion of covid-19.

The individual Healthcare worker is encouraged to contact the local Department of Health and/ or the CDC for guidance and information about vaccines.

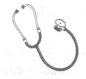

CHAPTER 12

EMOTIONAL AND PSYCHOLOGICAL EFFECTS OF DISASTERS

"Death is swallowed up in victory. Where O death is your victory, where O death is your sting"?

(1 Cor. 15:54b-55)

"According to the National Institute of Mental Health, 26.2% of the United States (US) population will experience a mental disorder within a given year, with 22.3% of those (5.8% of the US population) diagnosed as severely ill". (The Official Newsletter of the Central United States Earthquake Consortium, vol.15, No1; Winter, 20011).

http://www.ndu.edu/centercounter/index/htm).

Following the Terrorists' attacks on September 11, 2001, one could conclude that "fear and panic maybe as important to the terrorists as injury and death." (Center for Counter Proliferation Research National Defense University.

http://www.ndu.edu/centercounter/index/htm).

Four airlines with two planes crashed into the World Trade Center in New York City and one into the Pentagon in Washington, DC, the fourth in rural Pennsylvania. There were also two anthrax cases, in Florida, Robert

Stevens and Ernesto Blanco and the two deaths in Washington, DC, Joseph Curseen and Thomas Morris Jr.

Responding to this "Thomas Glass and Monica Spana suggest ["a bioterrorist attack is likely to produce a climate of grave uncertainty and insecurity, as has been the case in historic epidemics, and the general public will try to make sense of the experience of sudden widespread disease"]. Thomas Glass, Monica Schock-Spana, "Bioterrorism and the people: how to vaccinate a city against panic", Clinical Infectious Diseases, vol. 34, No. 2 (15 January 2002) p. 221.

Other efforts to prevent public panic after the anthrax events in Washington, DC were reported, one by John Schwartz, "The Truth Hurts: Efforts to Calm the Nation's Fears Spin out of Control", The New York Times, 28 Oct, 2001; p.1.

As with many major catastrophes, much of the population may likely experience the Five Stages of Grief.

https://www.psycom.net/stages-of-grief

The Five Stages of Grief:

1. Denial – The first stage of grief is Denial. It is really the first of our reactions to any form of sudden loss. Depending on the relationship we share to the subject of our loss, the more our lives may be uprooted or altered. It is very common for people to try and initially deny the event in order to subconsciously avoid sadness, or the thought of pending mental struggles. People in denial often withdraw from their normal social behavior and become isolated. Denial has no set time-frame, or may never be felt at all. However, it is considered the first stage of grief.

2. Anger – The second stage of grief is Anger. People that are grieving often become upset with the person or situation which put them in their grief state. After all, their life could now be in complete disarray. The path of least resistance is anger as opposed to facing the consequences of a loss head on. In the case of death, the anger is often focused toward the deceased for leaving that person behind and unable to cope. Other times people become angry at themselves if they feel they could have done something more to stop the loss from happening.

3. Bargaining – The third stage of grief is Bargaining. This is when those who are grieving are reaching out to the universe to make the pain go away. It is actually very normal, and largely considered to be a sign that they are beginning to comprehend their situation. People will often try to make a deal, or promise to do anything, if the pain will be taken away.

4. Depression – The fourth stage of grief is Depression. Contrary to popular belief, depression is something that may take some time to develop. We often think we are depressed when a grief event first occurs, but there is usually a lot of shock and other emotions present before any real depression can set in. The signs of depression due to grief usually appear when a sense of finality is realized. This is not to be confused with clinical depression, which may be chronic. Depression due to grief is technically episodic, even though it may last for a lengthy period of time.

5. Acceptance – The fifth stage of grief is Acceptance. This is the point where the person experiencing grief no longer is looking backward to try and recover the life they once had with the deceased, or other cause of their grief episode. It is not to say that they no longer feel the vast array of emotions brought on by their grief, but they are ready to embrace the idea that they are reaching a new point in their lives. At this point, they are beginning to understand that there is a new beginning on the horizon.

Acceptance should not be confused with healing or recovering from the loss, since that would put an enormous amount of pressure on people experiencing grief. Acceptance is really the beginning of the real healing process. It is the point where recovery becomes about the person left behind, and not about the person being mourned.

The Milbank Quarterly- a Multidisciplinary Journal of populations health and health policy, vol. 82, No. 3, 2004 presents findings from the

Rand Corporation titled "Emotional and Behavioral Consequences of Bioterrorism: Planning a Public Health Response".

We have quoted liberally from this writing in an attempt to provide some guidance to the reader when the occasion for a response is called for.

Since 9-11-01 and Oct. 3, 2001, the U.S. Public Health System has received millions of dollars in response to these events.

Chemical, Biological, Radiological and Nuclear Explosives [CBRNE] can be weapons of mass destruction [WMD], also referred to as weapons of effect (WME) used by terrorist groups, domestic and foreign. Some organizations consider it a religious duty to acquire these weapons and target Americans [Lumpskin, 2001, The Associated Press; Silmore Commission Reports, 1999, 2000, 2001, 2002].

In addition to death and destruction, considerable financial losses, significant emotional and behavioral consequences will occur, hence the designations as weapons of mass effect. Terrorism from CBRNE (basically Bioterrorism) differs from conventional terrorism such as hijacking on bombing as shown by the following from the Milbank Quarterly Report:

TABLE 1

Differences between Bioterrorism and Other forms of Terrorism

	Bioterrorism	**Other Forms**
Speed at which attack results	Delayed	Immediate
Site of attack	Unknown	Specific
Knowledge of attack scope or boundaries	Unknown	Usually well understood
Distribution of affected patients	multiple areas Concentrated areas	human to human transmission
First responders	Physicians, Nurses	Police, Fire, EMS
Isolation/quarantine	Required for transmissible disease	Not usually necessary
Medical interventions	antibiotics, vaccines antidotes	Trauma, first aid

An often asked question is which event in the District of Columbia resulted in most of the *emotional and behavioral changes: events of 911, the anthrax letters of* October 2001 or the *sniper events?*

Each individual will make that determination for themselves.

A major public health concern is the public's response to a bioterrorist event. What will be the demands on the health system by the worried well, those individuals without any apparent organic etiology for their symptoms? [Bartholomew, Wessely, Brit. Town of Psychiatry 180: 300-6, 2002].

The Sarin gas attack in Tokyo 1995 and other past events the US Department of Defense estimates a CBRNE attack would result in five psychological causalities for every one physical casualty. Emotional responses range from fear and anxiety to full blown psychiatric disorder.

Emotional – Post-Traumatic Stress Disorder (PTSD) and less severe generalized distress anxiety.

Behavioral – Seeking medical services, an increase in use of alcohol, tobacco and illicit drugs.

The Past Terrorist Events listed below were taken from an article in the Washington Post Newspaper, Friday July 8, 2005.

Past Terrorist Events

Date	City	Country	Facility	Type of Attack	Deaths
02-26-93	New York	USA	World Trade Center	Car Bomb	6
10-12-00	Aden	Yemen	USS Cole	Bomb	17
09-11-01	New York/ DC/PA	USA	World Trade Center/ Pentagon/PA	Planes	2,973
04-95	Oklahoma City	USA	Federal Building	Bomb	200
3-95	Tokyo	Japan	Subway	Gas	13
10-02	Florida/ Wash. DC/ MD/VA	USA	Random Sites	Sniper	5

Outbreaks of Severe Acute Respiratory Syndrome (SARS) 2003, the early days of HIV/AIDS and the Nuclear Meltdown at 3-mile Island, Pennsylvania (1979), offer comparative psychological events. Due to bioterrorism, the uncertainty of exposure may exist.

Literature review revealed little empirical information about the emotional and behavioral consequences of bioterrorism. Empirical data from other studies in the trauma field (Norris {n}) provided some guidance to help predict these consequences.

{n} pubmed.ncbi.nim.nih.gov/1619095/, Epidemiology of Trauma,

F. H. Norris, J. Consult Clin. Psychol. 1992 60(3):409-18.

A. Direct Victims (injury trauma).
B. General Public – Exposure commonly via media, TV, radio, newspapers.
C. First Responders.
D. Vulnerable populations – those who may be more susceptible to emotional and behavioral consequences, children with pre-existing psychological problems, pre-existing psychological problems, physical disabilities and drug dependent individual.

Uncertainty about exposure to an agent is likely to increase fear and anxiety. This uncertainty may occur among individually with low levels of exposure in the early phase, and possibly for months or years (example: Radiological Effects from a dirty bomb).

Depending upon the event, traditional first responders may be Fire/EMS/Police and healthcare personnel (SARS), thus the highest mortalities could be in Health Care workers if a covert Bioterrorist event were to occur. Before 9-11-01 the Oklahoma City bombing event of April 1995 was the only study I could find, documenting post-traumatic stress symptoms in individuals who did not hear, see or feel, the explosion.

After 9-11-01 a range or emotional and behavioral reactions were noted country wide.

Some surveys found a decrease in the prevalence of more severe emotional distress reactions in the general public, (Silver et.al, Stein et al. 2004) but also noted behavioral changes such as increase in use of cigarettes, alcohol, and marijuana in New York (Vlahov et al. 2004) and an increase in suboptimal doses of antiretroviral therapies in HIV positive men in New York City (Hepatitis et.al. 2003).

Several studies found a higher level of anxiety among the general population. (See WHO reference below). Many of the emotional and behavioral reactions and fears of contagion reported by health care workers in response to SARS were like those noted a decade ago in the early phases of HIV/AIDS. Table 5 focuses on vulnerable populations.

Table 5: Psychological Consequences Measured in Vulnerable Population (The Milbank Quarterly vol., 82 No 3, 2004)

Event	Vulnerable Populations
Intentional Mass Violence/Conventional Terrorism	
Bombing of Murrah Federal Building, Oklahoma City, April 1995	Almost 20% of sixth-grade students in a town approximately 100 miles from Oklahoma City reported bomb, difficulty functioning two years after the attack. Clinical need assessment conducted with sixth to the students seven weeks after the bombing found that posttraumatic stress symptoms were significantly females, children who knew someone injured or killed children who reported watching more bombings on television news coverage. Seven weeks following the attack, a majority of children from Oklahoma City area reported fear that a friend or someone from their family would be hurt and reported being afraid; 40% felt helpless. Fear, arousal and dissociation time of the bombing was the strongest predictor of posttraumatic stress symptoms, more important the exposure, relationship to direct victims, bomb-related television viewing, and continued safety concerns.
Terrorist attacks on World Trade Center (WTC) and Pentagon, September 2001.	Three to five days after the attack, almost one-third children ages five to 18 in households experience emotional stress symptoms, and 42% discussed them with their parents.

One to two months after the attacks, parents in 48% households with children reported that at least on household was upset by the attacks on Sept. 11. The percent of these children had trouble sleeping; 30% irritable, grouchy, or easily upset; and 27% were fearing separation from their parents.

Twenty-two percent of parents living in lower Manhattan surveys five to eight weeks after the attacks reported their children had received some form of counseling their experience after the WTC attack. More than counseling was delivered in schools.

Within two months following the attacks, an increased for drug and alcohol treatment was found among the with preexisting psychological problems in 13 major cities.

Significant increase was reported in children's visits health clinics for acute and posttraumatic stress response other anxiety disorders at military treatment facility 50 miles of Washington D.C. for five months after compared with same period in the previous two years.

Survey of drug users conducted between one and four following the attacks found significant anxiety, and sadness; increase in drug use was as common as recent drug use.

The World Health Organization (WHO) has listed a number of "key facts" relating to mental Health in emergencies. "Almost all people affected by emergencies will experience psychological distress, which for most people will improve over time. Depression tends to be more common in women than men, and more common as people get older.

People with severe mental disorders are especially vulnerable during emergencies and need access to mental health and other basic needs.

Social problems, e.g., poverty and discrimination, interact with the mental health issues relating to increased anxiety due to lack of information. People with severe mental disorders can be especially vulnerable during and after emergencies, and they need access to basic needs and clinical care. Clinical care should be provided by, or under the supervision of Psychiatrists, Psychologists or Psychiatric Nurses.

Mental health should also be a component of National Disaster Preparedness Plans". https://www.who.int/news-room/fact-sheets/detail/mental-health-in-emergencies.

The Substance Abuse and Mental Health Services Administration (SAMHSA) provides communities and responders with behavioral health resources that help them prepare, respond and recover from disasters. https://www.samhsa.gov/disaster-preparedness.

In an article from Rick Nauert, PhD, the John Hopkins University Researcher states "more attention should be devoted to triaging and managing those identified as having mental disorders. These can include conditions such as addictions, Bipolar disorder, Dementia, Post Traumatic Distress Disorder [PTSD] and Schizophrenia. Many of the mentally ill are dependent on caretakers and are not fully capable of making sound decisions. One study found that 22 percent of Hurricane Katrina survivors who had pre-existing mental disorders faced limited or had terminated treatment after the disaster. Because of the demand, many licensed professionals may be unavailable immediately after a disaster so first responders, other healthcare workers, volunteers, should be trained to provide Psychological First Aid.

Policies may need to be made in catastrophic situations where-by legally trained personnel may provide certain sedatives as was the case in New

York City immediately after the September 11 Terrorist Attack". https://psycentral.com/news/2011/05/24/disaster-plans-should-include-those-with-mental-illness/26432.html (Last updated: 8 Aug 2018).

Caplan, in Preventive Psychiatry, 1964, referred to "an acute RESPONSE to a trauma, disaster or other critical incident as a Psychological Crisis, where-in one's usual coping mechanisms have failed". He further noted that Critical Incident Stress Management (CISM) which is "an integrated, multi-component strategic crisis intervention system is the most widely used system world wide".

Another important principle in addressing this issue is Psychological First Aid (PFA), defined by Dr. George S. Everly Jr., PhD, "as a compassionate and supportive presence designed to mitigate acute distress and assess the need for continued mental health care. It can serve as the platform on which more advanced individual and group crisis and disaster mental health intervention can be built".

"PFA is NOT THERAPY nor a substitute for THERAPY but a variation on the theme of Crisis Intervention."

Everly, G.S., Jr. & Mitchell, J.T. (2008). Integrative Crisis Intervention and Disaster Mental Health. Ellicott City, MD, Chevron.

CISM and PFA should work collaboratively in providing the continuum of care needed the Psychological Crisis.

As a means of measuring Health and Disability the World Health Organization (WHO) has developed a Disability Assessment Schedule which addresses 6 Domains of Functioning:

WHODAS 2.0: Cognition, Mobility, Self-care, Getting along, Life Activities and Participation.

https://www.who.int/classifications/icf/whodasii/en/

What about the relationship between Spirituality and Religion in general health and mental health?

It is generally accepted by some that a large percentage of the population in the United States (US) practices or is related to some form of Religion. [R]

Some are not and consider themselves atheists or agnostics. (a,a)

The major Religious Ideologies in the US when health issues are concerned are Buddhism, Catholicism, Hinduism, Islam, Judaism and Protestantism. (B, C, H). The most common form of outward expression of participation with each of these Groups is prayer. [P]

With respect to response to a terrorist event, viz, bereavement, each of these Ideologies does so according to their beliefs. [b]

Pragmatically, Spiritualism is difficult to measure and many Practitioners are not formally trained in addressing this topic. [sp]

"The Joint Commission, which evaluates and accredits healthcare organizations in the US, mandates that Practitioners conduct an initial, brief assessment about Spirituality but has not developed specific Guidelines for a comprehensive assessment. [*]

The 4 key principles of the Joint commission are respect, honesty, fairness and integrity. Overlooking spirituality leaves patients feeling disconnected from the healthcare system and the clinicians trying to care for them". [*]

(a,a) Newport F, Religious Identity: http://news.gallop.com/poll/122075/Religious-Identy-States Differ-Wide ly.aspx. Last assessed4/3/2018.
(a,a) Newport F, Estimating:
httpsl/news.gallop.com/poll/2070/Estimating-Americans-Workshops-

Behavior.aspx. Last assessed 4/3/2018.

[R] Mayers C, Johnson D, Spirituality...Implicit Religion, 2008;11(3):255-264
[H,C,D] NetCE.com/MD, vol. 145, No. 5, 2019 Course #91982, Role of Spirituality, page 9,10.

[P] Clarke TC, et al, Natl Health Stat Report 2015;79:1-15

b Care....http://www.uphs.upen.edu/pastoral/resd/diversity_points.html. Last assessed 4/3/2018

[S] Bremault –Phillips S, Olson J.et al. Integrating Spirituality as a key component of patient care. Religions, 2015;6(2):476-498

[S] Larsen KM, Rinkel M, What does religion...Relig Spiritual Soc. work mean to a racially diverse... 2016;35(3);200-221.

* https:/www.jointcommission.org>standards-faqs-pr

Inherent in the thought processes of many in Western Civilizations as a factor in Religion is the concept of The Four Last Things, Death, Judgement, Heaven and Hell. (tf)

The Roman Catholic Religion believes there is a domain between Heaven and Hell called Purgatory.

While accepting the fact that some segments of a civilized society do not accept the concept of "sin", the Roman Catholic Church also puts forth the premise of the Seven Deadly Sins, Pride, Covetousness. Lust, Anger, Gluttony, Envy and Sloth.

To counter these "sins" are the Seven Virtues, Humility, Liberality, Chasity, Meekness, Temperance, Brotherly Love and Diligence. [D]

Also, inherent here-in are the cultural competencies of the various populations in the United States. This includes cultural sensitivity, cultural knowledge and cultural skills, which are inter-connected and determine in part, their response to major disaster, death and bereavement (cc, db).

(tf) en.wikipedia.org/wiki/Four-last-things.
(cc) Artiff KM, Beng KS, Cultural health...Aust J Rural Health, 2006;14(1):2-8.
(db). HealthCare Chaplaincy.http://www.healthcarechaplaincy.org/userimaages/doc/cultural, Documentary.pdf. last assessed 8/14/2018.
(db). Penn Med Pastoral Care.
http://www.uphs.upenn.edu/pastoral/resed.diversity points.html. Last assesses 8/14/2018.
[D] Manual of Prayers, 3rd Edition, Pontifical North American College, p 48, nacrome@aool.com.

When this Book was initially written, Covid-19 and Monkey Pox (although a known disease) were not illnesses which required world health responses at the time.

Likewise, injuries and deaths from Gun Shot wounds, while long being health care concerns, were not at endemic proportions as they are now in 2022 in this country.

As with all of the events discussed in previous Chapters, the Healthcare Provider should follow the directions of their local Departments of Health when responding to these events.

AFTERWORD

When I received the copyright for the title of this Book on December 27, 2009, I was sure I would have it finished and published much earlier.

As I stated in the Foreword, in my opinion, the current state of world affairs, almost mandates a Book of this kind, as at any time, healthcare providers may be called upon to respond to an All-Hazards Emergency, presenting in a trice as a Derecho.

In the past 2 years, over 6 million people have died world-wide from the novel virus covid-19. On July 23, 2022, the World Health Organization has declared Monkey pox, a viral disease, with over 16,500 cases in 68 countries, as a Global Emergency; however, in 2023, that designation has been removed, and Monkey pox is now referred to as M-pox.

In the United States of America, there have been over 40,000 deaths from gunshot violence in the past few years, including many children in our schools, and in my opinion, this country's pandemic.

When a young Black boy cannot ring a door bell without the risk of being shot, or a young White female cannot make a wrong turn into a drive-way, without the risk of being shot and killed, when a 6 year- old boy shoots his teacher, something is terribly wrong with our society.

According to the CDC, "All fire arm deaths in 2021were 48,830, with 14.7 deaths per 100,000 population".

National Vital Statistics System-Mortality Data (2021) via CDC WONDER. [1]

> The Author does not wish to imply, in any way, that he is an expert, of any sort!

The book is intended to be a reference source, for any healthcare provider, in the broad area of Emergency Preparedness.

Because the world is so "closely connected" now, transportation and internet wise, perhaps this Book can be a tool to help us become better prepared as healthcare providers for these events…but what can we do to help us truly believe and live by "The Golden Rule…the principle of treating others as one wants to be treated"?

GR https://www.wikipedia.org.wiki>GoldenRule.

[1] cdc.gov/nchs/faststsats/injuries.htm.

Questions from Essentials of Emergency Preparedness:
A Primer for Healthcare Providers.

1. All-Hazardous preparation includes which of the following:

    A. Rapid detection
    B. Surge capacity
    C. Mass containment strategy
    D. Effective communication
    E. All of the above

2. With regards to disaster planning, which of the following terms does not apply?

    A. Preparedness
    B. Response
    C. Recovery
    D. Data analysis
    E. Mitigation

3. Which of the following will most likely contribute to a successful disaster response?

    A. Interoperable and redundant communication.
    B. Having a CEO or COO acting as the Incident Commander.
    C. Strict scene and hospital security.
    D. A and C.

4. Which of the following positions must be filled in the Incident Command (ICS) system?

    A. Safety Officer.
    B. Public Relations Officer.
    C. Logistics Officer.
    D. Incident Commander.
    E. Planning Officer.

5. In the ICS structure, which position is responsible for transportation and communication?

    A. Planning Officer.
    B. Safety Officer.
    C. Logistics Officer.
    D. Public Information Officer.

6. The only person (s) in the Incident Command System who can abort a Training exercise or active participation in a suspected Terrorist event is the:

    A. Safety Officer.
    B. Incident Commander.
    C. Public Information Officer.
    D. Administrative Officer.
    E. A and B.

7. Which one of the following is one of the 5 major functional elements of the ICS?

    A. Law Enforcement.
    B. HAZMAT/Decontamination.
    C. Search and rescue.
    D. Planning.
    E. Medical care.

8. The Federal statue prohibiting use of the military in civilian law enforcement is which of the following?

    A. The Maritime Transportation Security Act.
    B. The Posse Comitatus Act.
    C. The Patriot Act.
    D. The Robert T. Stafford Emergency Assistance Act.

9. The Robert T. Stafford Relief and Emergency Assistance Act in 1958:

   A. Highlights the responsibility of specific federal agencies during a terrorism event.
   B. Designates consequence management to the Federal Bureau of Investigation during a terrorism event.
   C. Requires the Federal Emergency Management Agency (FEMA) to reimburse 90% of expenses accrued in investigation and death from a terrorism event, to the investigating agency.
   D. All of the above.
   E. C only.

10. With regards to disaster planning, which of the following terms does not apply?

    A. Preparedness.
    B. Response.
    C. Recovery.
    D. Degradation.
    E. Mitigation.

11. Which of the following will most likely contribute to a successful disaster response?

    A. Interoperable and redundant communications.
    B. Having the COO or the CEO acting as the Incident Commander.
    C. Strict scene and hospital security.
    D. A and C.
    E. Requesting the local Media to ask for blood donations

12. With respect to Risk Communications to ease public concern about a looming biological event, which of the following should be included in the message?

   A. The risk is low.
   B. The illness is treatable.
   C. The disease is not easily transmitted from person to person.
   D. Symptoms are easily recognizable.
   E. All of the above.

13. All-Hazardous preparation includes which of the following?

   A. Rapid detection.
   B. Surge capacity.
   C. Mass containment strategy.
   D. Effective communication.
   E. All of the above.

14. Which of the following is most appropriate in the prehospital phase of a mass casualty disaster response?

   A. Allowing scene responders to decide for themselves when to rest.
   B. Assuring the safety of responders, before casualties, as the first priority.
   C. Continuing search and rescue operations until all victims are found.
   D. Transport of all living casualties from the scene directly to the nearest hospital.

15. The CDC categorization of Category A Bio-terrorism agents includes which of the following?

   A. Easily disseminated and/or transmitted from person to person.
   B. Results in high morbidity and mortality.
   C. May cause public panic and social disruption.
   D. Require special action for public health preparedness.
   E. All of the above.

16. Anthrax is a gram-positive rod. Which of the following is NOT a characteristic?

    A. Encapsulated.
    B. Non-motile.
    C. Non-hemolytic.
    D. Non-spore forming.
    E. Box-car shape.

17. True or false.
    The Anthrax spores can remain viable for decades.

18. Which of the following is the pathway by which Anthrax attacks an individual?

    A. Edema factor +lethal factor = protective antigen.
    B. Protective antigen+ edema factor=lethal factor.
    C. Lethal factor+ protective antigen= lethal toxin.
    D. D Edema factor+ protective antigen = edema toxin.
    E. Some other pathway.

19. True or False
    The presence of Anthrax spores from a nasal swap indicates the individual has inhalational Anthrax.

20. The term which this statement best defines, "Animal borne disease that can be spread to humans, and from humans to humans" is:

    A. Enzootic.
    B. Epizootic
    C. Prevalence.
    D. Zoonosis.

21. The CDC estimates the number of cases, hospitalizations, and deaths from food borne illness are:

    A. 50,000, 150,000, 5,000.
    B. 48 million, 128,000, 3,000.
    C. 75,000, 125,000, 2,000.
    D. 900,000, 325,000, 2,500.

22. The recommended treatment for Noro virus illness, the primary cause of foodborne illness in the USA is?

    A. Vancomycin.
    B. Ampicillin.
    C. Rest and keep hydrated.
    D. Steroids.

23. Which of the following is the causative agent for Botulism?

    A. Yersinia pestis.
    B. Clostridium perfringens.
    C. Clostridium botulinum.
    D. Varicella.

24. Which of the following is not associated with Botulism?

    A. Diplopia.
    B. Dysarthria.
    C. Dysphonia.
    D. Diaphoresis
    E. Dysphagia.

25. Which of the following is NOT recommended for infants under age 12 months because of possible association with Botulism?

    A. Granulated sugar.
    B. Chocolates.
    C. Peaches.
    D. Honey.

26. The term "Rice water" is used to describe the diarrhea seen in which illness?

    A. Shigella.
    B. Salmonellosis.
    C. Cholera.
    D. Enterohemorrhagic coli.

27. Individuals with untreated Cholera have been known to lose what percent of body weight in fluids.

    A. 2%.
    B. 5%.
    C. 7%.
    D. 10%.

28. Which individual demonstrated that human sewage contamination was the most probable disease vector for Cholera?

    A. Robert Koch.
    B. Edward Jenner.
    C. Luis Pasteur
    D. John Snow.

29. Which individual identified the organism Vibrio cholera which caused Cholera?

    A. Edward Jenner.
    B. Robert Koch.
    C. John Snow.
    D. Luis Pasteur.

30. Which President of the United States of America died from cholera?

    A. James Madison.
    B. James Polk.
    C. Woodrow Wilson.
    D. James Buchanan.

31. Match the following mosquitoes with the disease they are commonly associated with.

    A. Anopheles   ____Dengue
    B. Aedes   ____Malaria
    C. Culex   ____West Nile
                     ____St. Louis Equine Encephalitis
                     ____Yellow Fever
                     ____Zika

32. True or False.
    Immunity to all 4 of the Dengue Serotypes is obtained when infected by any one of the Serotypes.

33. Globally there are now recorded how many cases of Dengue world-wide?

    A. 500.000.
    B. 2.5 million.
    C. 3.5 billion.
    D. 3.5 million.

34. With regards to Humoral Immunity, which type of cells destroys foreign antigens?

    A. White blood cells.
    B. B cells.
    C. Lymphocytes.
    D. T cells.

35. The Dengue vaccine, Dengvaxia, by Sanofi Pasteur is recommended for those living in endemic areas who are aged:

    A. 6 months to 7 years.
    B. 9 years to 16 years.
    C. 15 years to 40 years.
    D. 65 years and older.

36. Although there is no specific treatment for Dengue, aggressive supportive care has reduced mortality rates to:

    A. Less than 10%.
    B. Less than 15%.
    C. Less than 20%.
    D. Less than 1%.

37. With regards to Cellular Immunity, which type of cells destroy foreign antigens?

    A. White blood cells.
    B. Lymphocytes.
    C. B cells.
    D. T cells.

38. The host for the Ebola virus is thought to be:

    A. The Civet Cat.
    B. Aegis aegypti mosquito.
    C. The Fruit Bat.
    D. A Camel.
    E. The Deer Mouse.

39. The Ebola virus possibly gains entrance to a human host via:

    A. Inhalation.
    B. The oral-fecal route.
    C. The mucous membranes, bodily fluids.
    D. A and C.
    E. Some other route.

40. Most of the cases of Ebola during the outbreak in West Africa in 2014-2016 were:

    A. 6 months to age 2 years.
    B. Ages 2-5 years.
    C. Ages 10- 25 years.
    D. Ages 15 to 44 years.
    E. Ages 45 years and older.

41. The usual onset of symptoms in Ebola is:

    A. 2-3 days.
    B. 5-7 days
    C. 8-12 days.
    D. 12-21 days.

42. True or False.
    A person who dies from Ebola should be embalmed as soon as possible?

43. Exposure to Aflatoxin is associated with an increased risk of which cancer?

    A. Lung.
    B. Liver.
    C. Stomach,
    D. Bladder.

44. Which of the following is recommended as a prophylactic and therapeutic measure for persons exposed to Aflatoxins?

    A. Vitamin A
    B. Vitamin C.
    C. Vitamin D.
    D. Vitamin E.

45. Which of the following is an emerging yeast infection that is multi-drug resistant?

    A. Candida albicans.
    B. Candida auris.
    C. Candida aspergillus.
    D. Candida esophagitis.

46. Candida auris, an emerging yeast infection is best treated by treated with?

    A. Antibiotics.
    B. Antivirals.
    C. Defoliants.
    D. Echinocandins.

47. The illness which may result from an infection with as few as 10 organisms` is?

    A. Tularemia.
    B. Q Fever.
    C. Dengue.
    D. West Nile virus.

48. Which of the following organisms is the causative agent for Q Fever?

    A. Escherichia coli.
    B. Yersinia pestis.
    C. Rickettsia felis.
    D. Coxiella burnetii.

49. Chronic Q Fever may be associated with which of the following?

    A. Hemolytic anemia.
    B. Epididymitis/Orchitis.
    C. Myocarditis.
    D. Osteomyelitis.
    E. All of the above.

50. A process by which two or more different strains of a virus, e.g., Influenza A, or two more different viruses, combine to form a new subtype, having a mixture of the surface antigens of the two or more original strains` is called _____?

51. The natural mutation over time of known strains of Influenza A, B an C viruses which may lead to loss of immunity to those particular strains' is called_____?

52. The parasite which is the most common cause of death is Malaria is:

    A. Plasmodium ovale.
    B. Plasmodium falciparum.
    C. Plasmodium malariae.
    D. Plasmodium vivax.

53. True of False.
The gold standard for diagnosis of Malaria is the microscopic examination of the cells which show the parasite.

54. The transmissible agent responsible for infection in Mad Cow Disease, Chronic Wasting Disease, Creutzfeldt- Jakob Disease (CJD) and the Variant Creutzfeldt-Jakob (vCJD) is the _____ ?

55. The ability to provide adequate medical evaluation and care during events that exceed the limits of the normal medical infrastructure is _____?

56. The ability to response to an increased volume of patients with an adequate number of hospital beds, personnel, medical supplies and equipment is_____?

57. The ability to manage patients requiring specialized evaluation and medical care is _____ _____?

58. The organism responsible for the Plague is?

    A. Culex pipiens.
    B. Vaccinia.
    C. Yersenia pestis.
    D. Aedes species.

59. What is the new call number for suicide prevention?

    A. 211.
    B. 611.
    C. 811.
    D. 988.

60. True or False?
Primary Pneumonic Plague is transmissible from human to human and from animal to human.

61. Which of the following diseases may be associated with buboes (Infected femoral-inguinal lymph nodes)?

    A. Chlamydia.
    B. Chancroid.
    C. Plague.
    D. Tuberculosis.
    E. All of the above.

62. The Deer Mouse is the Primary Host for the virus which causes which disease?

    A. West Nile virus.
    B. Dengue Fever.
    C. Zika
    D. Sin Nombre, (Hanta Virus).

63. Which of the following has been known to cause death from massive multi-organ failure within 36 hours?

    A. Botulism.
    B. Prion infection.
    C. Nerve Gas toxicity.
    D. Ricin.

64. Small pox is caused by which of the following viruses?

    A. Varicella.
    B. Vaccinia.
    C. Variola.
    D. Filovirus.

65. True or False?
Vaccinia, the live virus used to vaccinate to prevent Small pox can cause Small pox.

66. The Nations largest supply of medical counter measures in a public health emergency, severe enough to cause local suppliesto be depleted is the_____?

67. With respect to Chemical Agents, a CHEMPACK in a Hospital formulary may include?

    A. Mark-1 Kits.
    B. Atropine Sulfate Injectors.
    C. Diazepam Injectors.
    D. Pralidoxime.
    E. All of the above.

68. The role of Pralidoxime (2-Pam) in treating Nerve Gas Incidents` is to:

    A. Block the effects of excess acetylcholine.
    B. Reduce severity of convulsions.
    C. Prevents vomiting and diarrhea.
    D. Reactivates acetylcholine esterase.

69. Lead levels in children of what number below indicates a high probability of behavior problems and learning disabilities?

    A. 2ug/dl.
    B. 4 ug/dl.
    C. 8ug/dl.
    D. 12 ug/dl.

70. What does the following acronym stand for?

    S
    L
    U
    D
    G
    E

71. What does the following acronym stand for?

    D
    U
    M
    B
    E
    L
    S

72. The most toxic Nerve Agent available in the West is?

    A. Sarin.
    B. Soman.
    C. Tabun.
    D. Vx.

73. Which of these agents is more toxic than Vx?

    A. Anthrax
    B. Botulinum.
    C. Sarin.
    D. Tabun.

74. In children, which symptom is least useful in diagnosing Nerve Agent toxicity?

    A. Tachycardia.
    B. Hypertension.
    C. Tachycardia,
    D. Miosis.

75. All of the following are muscarinic effects of Nerve Agent Toxicity except?

    A. Bronchorrhea.
    B. Miosis.
    C. Salivation.
    D. Sweating.
    E. All of the above are.

76. All of the following are nicotinic effects of Nerve Agent Toxicity except?

    A. Tachycardia.
    B. Hypertension.
    C. Muscle twitching.
    D. Diarrhea.

77. The name of the radioactive agent associated with the Dirty Bomb, Radio-active Diversion Device (RDD) Reported in Brazil in1987 was:

    A. Americum 241.
    B. Cesium 137.
    C. Cobalt 60.
    D. Irridium 192.

78. Which of the following has been proven effective for treating ingested Cesium 137?

    A. Activated Charcoal.
    B. Ipicac.
    C. Prussian blue.
    D. Some other agent.

79. Match the following names with the event they are associated with.

    A. Otto Hahn.   ____ Nuke Map
    B. Lise Meitner.   ____ Nuclear Physicist
    C. Robert Oppenheimer   ____ Atomic Bomb
    D. Alex Wellerstein.   ____ Dynamite.
    E. Alfred Nobel

80. Match the following chemical agents, alphabets, with their corresponding number.

    A. Mustard Gas, (Lewisite).   ____ 1 Riot Control.
    B. Phosgene.   ____ 2 Blistering.
    C. Sarin   ____ 3 Blood.
    D. Cyanide   ____ 4 Nerve Agent.
    E. Tear Gas.   ____ 5 Choking.

81. Which statement(s) is/are true?

    A. The KKK originated in South in opposition to Reconstruction.
    B. The KKK in 1915 was a response to the Labor movement.
    C. The KKK was against the Civil Rights Movement.
    D. The KKK developed in 3 waves in the USA.
    E. Only C above.
    F. All of the above are correct.

82. The chain of Survival in Emergency Cardiac Care consists of all of the following, except?

    A. Immediate recognition and activation of the response system.
    B. Early CPR.
    C. Rapid Defibrillation.
    D. Integrated post-cardiac arrest care.
    E. All of the above.

83. When considering surgery for individuals who have sustained acute radiological injuries, the optimal time to operate is?

    A. Within the first 6 to 12 hours.
    B. Within the first 12 to 24 hours.
    C. Within the first 36 to 48 hours, if not, 6 weeks later.
    D. Within the first 36 to 48 hours, if not, 3 to 4 weeks later.
    E. Each case has to be determined on an individual basis.

84. The greatest Risk Factor for recovery by an individual from the effects of an Acute Radiation Injury is?

    A. Absolute Neutrophil Count (ANC)>100,000/uL.
    B. Absolute Neutrophil Count (ANC) <100,000/uL.
    C. Total Lymphocyte Count of >3,000 cells/uL.
    D. Platelet Count >400,000.

85. When a persons loved one dies, he or she is likely to experience:

    A. 4 Stages of sadness.
    B. 4 Stages of loneness.
    C. 5 Stages of grief.
    D. Some other emotional experiences.

86. In Acute Radiation injuries, which phase of the Gastrointestinal Syndrome presents as severe nausea, vomiting, cramps and diarrhea?

    A. Latent phase.
    B. Manifest illness phase.
    C. Prodromal phase.
    D. Recovery phase.

87. The common vector for Ebola and Marburg Fever is the:

    A. African Rat.
    B. The Fruit Bat.
    C. Aedes albopictus Mosquito.
    D. Culex pipiens mosquito.

88. Which of the following poisons cause Acrodynia (Pink Disease) in children?

    A. Lead.
    B. Mercury.
    C. Thallium.
    D. Arsenic.

89. The following are common animal pet diseases.

    A. Hookworm.
    B. Ringworm.
    C. Roundworm.
    D. Psittacosis (Parrott Fever).
    E. Lyme.
    F. All are.

90. Match the following types of explosions with the injuries caused.

A. Primary   _____ Radiation, Dirty Bomb.

B. Secondary   _____ Burns, Inhalation.

C. Tertiary   _____ Blunt trauma Crush injury.

D. Quaternary   _____Most common

E. Quinary   _____ Hollow viscus

91. Each of the following is a phase of the Emergency Management Cycle except?

A. Prevention.
B. Response.
C. Triage.
D. Recovery.
E. Mitigation

92. The 3 most common chemicals causing illness are?

A. Chlorine.
B. Phosgene.
C. Cyanide.
D. Anhydrous Ammonia.
E. A, B and D.

93. Rabbits are most commonly infected in the USA with which disease?

A. Tularemia.
B. Lyme disease.
C. Plague.
D. West Nile virus.

94. Match the following Presidential Directive with their action.

   A. PD 5   ____ NIMS
   B. PD 8   ____ Bioterrorism
   C. PD 10   ____Public Health
   D. PD 20   ____ National Preparedness
   E. PD 21   ____ Continuity of Federal Gov

95. The vaccine for Hepatitis B is an example of which type of vaccine?

   A. Inactivated (killed).
   B. Live, attenuated.
   C. Conjugated.
   D. Subunit.

96. The type of vaccine for young children who do not generate a strong response to a certain antigen is?

   A. Live, attenuated.
   B. Subunit
   C. Conjugated.
   D. Some other vaccine.

97. FDA recommendations for treating covid- 19 are all except?

   A. Remdesivir.
   B. Invermectin.
   C. Paxlovid.
   D. Baricitnib.

98. Patients who are receiving chemotherapy or radiation therapy, should, or should not, receive the annual Influenza vaccine?

99. 100. Match the following "sins" with the "virtues".

A. Covetousness	___ Brotherly love
B. Anger.	___ Meekness
C. Lust.	___ Humility
D. Envy.	___ Diligence
E. Gluttony.	___ Liberality
F. Sloth.	___ Chasity
G. Pride	___ Temperance

101 .Match the following Diseases in Column A to the Vaccines in Column B. (5 points)

A. Column A	Column B
B. Covid-19	___Shingrix
C. Dengue	___Arexvy, Abrsvd
D. Ebola	___Novavax
E. Pneumonia	___Dengvaxia
F. Respiratory Syncytial Virus (RSV)	___PCV15,PCV20
G. Shingles	___rVSV-ZEBOV (Ervebo)

Answers:

1	E. All of above.
2	D. Data analysis
3	A and C
4	D
5	C
6	E and B.
7	D. planning.
8	B
9	C only
10	D. Degradation.
11	D. A and C.
12	E. all
13	E. all
14	B
15	E. All of above.
16	D
17	True
18	C
19	FALSE
20	D. Zoonosis
21	B
22	C
23	C
24	D
25	D
26	C
27	D
28	B
29	B
30	B
31	A. Anopheles B_Dengue

B. Aedes   A_Malaria
C. Culex   C_West Nile Virus
                  C_St. Louis Virus
                  B_Yellow Fever
                  B_Zika

32	FALSE
33	B
34	B
35	B
36	D
37	D
38	C
39	C
40	D
41	C
42	FALSE
43	B
44	A
45	B
46	D
47	A
48	D
49	E
50	Antigenic shift
51	Antigenic drift
52	B
53	TRUE
54	Prion
52	Medical Surge
56	Surge Capacity
57	Surge Capability
58	C
59	D. 988

60	TRUE	
61	E	
62	D	
63	D	
64	C	
65	Fales	
66	Strategic National Stockpile (SNS)	
67	E	
68	D	
69	D	
70	Salivation	Diarrhea
	Lacrimation	Urination
	Urination	Miosis
	Defecation	Bronchorrhea
	Gastro intestinal	Emesis
	Emesis	Lacrimation
		Salivation
71		B
	E	
	L	
S		
72	D	
73	B	
74	D	
75	ALL ARE	
76	D	
	B. cesium -	
77	Cesium137	
78	C. Prussian Blue	
79	A.	D Nuke Map
	B	A, B Nuclear Physicist
	C	C Atomic Bomb
	D	E Dynamite

212

	E	
80	A	__E. Riot Control
	B	__A Blistering
	C	__D Blood
	D	__C -Nerve agent
	E	__ B Choking
81	F. All of the above	
82	E. All of the Above	
83	D	
84	B	
85	C	
86	C	
87	B	
88	B	
89	F	
90	A	____E Radiation, dirty Bomb
	B	____D Burns, inhalation
	C	____C Blunt trauma, crush injury
	D	____ B Most common injury, projectile
	E	____ A Hollow viscus, ear drum
91	C	
92	E	
93	A	
94	PD 5	____5 NIMS, Domestic incidents
	PD 8	10 Bioterrorism
	PD 10	_____8 National preparedness
	PD 20	_____20 Continuity of Federal government
	PD 21	_____21 Public Health
95	D	
96	C	
97	B	
98	Should	

99,100   A. Anger.   C_ Brotherly love

          B. Covetousness   E _Chasity

          C. Envy   G _Diligence

          D. Gluttony   F_ Humility

          E. Lust   B_ Liberality

          F. Pride   A_ Meekness

          G. Sloth   D_ Temperance

101   Match the following Diseases in Column A with the Vaccines
          in Column B. (Worth 5 points).

          A. Covid-19   _E_Shringrix

          B. Dengue   _F_Arexvy, Abrysvo

          C. Ebola   _A_Novavax

          D. Pneumonia   _B_Dengvexia

          E. Shingles   _D_PRV15, PRV20

          F. Respiratory Syncytia _C_rVSV-ZEBOV (Ervebo)
          Virus (RSV) l

Printed in the United States
by Baker & Taylor Publisher Services